Home Office Handbook - Ergonomic Solutions For Back Pain

How To Establish A Comfortable, Pain-Free Home Workspace

Dr. Susan Jameson, Chiropractor

Second Edition

COPYRIGHT

Home Office Handbook- Ergonomic Solutions for Back Pain

Copyright © 2025 by Dr. Susan Jameson

All rights reserved.

Second Edition: 2025

No part of this publication may be reproduced, stored in a retrieval system, or transmitted in any form or by any means—electronic, mechanical, photocopying, recording, or otherwise—without the prior written permission of the author, except in the case of brief quotations used in articles or reviews.

This book is intended for informational purposes only. It is not a substitute for professional medical advice, diagnosis, or treatment. Always consult with a qualified healthcare provider before making any changes to your healthcare or ergonomic setup.

Author: Dr. Susan Jameson, Chiropractor

Title: Home Office Handbook- Ergonomic Solutions for Back Pain

Subtitle: How To Create A Pain-Free, Comfortable Workspace

Print ISBN: 978-1-7640830-3-4

Published by: Better Back Solutions

National Library of Australia

Cataloging-in-Publication entry available upon request. Legal deposit compliant with the Copyright Act 1968 (Cth).

PRAISE FROM READERS

"Practical, easy-to-follow guidance for anyone who works long hours at a desk."

"Well organised, easy to read, and genuinely useful."

"I didn't know many of these solutions existed. I will definitely be trying some of them."

"Clear, realistic advice that makes an immediate difference — without needing expensive equipment."

"Backed by real ergonomic science and solid clinical experience."

"Helped me reduce daily back, neck, and arm discomfort by making simple, achievable adjustments."

"I learned about active sitting, a game changer for my back and neck."

"I changed my sitting posture and immediately felt the benefits."

Edition Note

This Second Edition of *Home Office Handbook – Ergonomic Solutions for Back Pain* has been updated to provide improved flow, refined language, and expanded ergonomic strategies for today's hybrid and remote work environments.

Chapters have been streamlined to remove repetition, transitions enhanced for smoother reading, and the latest posture and workspace research integrated to ensure this guide remains practical and relevant for modern professionals.

Table of Contents

Introduction	IX
1. The New Work Landscape	1
2. Taking Care of Your Back	6
3. Home Office Ergonomics	14
4. Ergonomic Chairs - The Heart Of Your Setup	24
5. Standing Desks: A Game-Changer In Back Care	30
6. Active Sitting Solutions and Dynamic Posture	38
7. Troubleshooting Your Ergonomic Setup	46
8. Saddle Seats: Ergonomic Seating Revolution	52
9. Kneeling Chairs To Reduce Back Pain	58
10. Stability Ball - A Versatile Tool For Back Pain Relief	63
11. Ergonomic Accessories	69
12. Keyboard Tray	71
13. Ergonomic Keyboard and Mouse	74
14. Wrist Pads	77
15. Document Holder	80
16. Headset	83

17.	Noise-Cancelling Headphones	86
18.	Footrest	89
19.	Anti-Fatigue Mat	92
20.	Posture Wedge	95
21.	Wobble Cushion	98
22.	Lumbar Cushion	100
23.	Conclusion - Living And Working In Alignment	104
Annotated Bibliography		105
Author		110
Also In This Series		111
Leave A Review		113

Introduction

Over the past few years, the way we work has changed dramatically. More people than ever are working from home, spending long hours at makeshift desks, kitchen tables, and even couches. While remote work has offered flexibility and freedom, it has also introduced a growing problem: back pain, neck, shoulder and arm pain.

As a chiropractor with years of clinical experience, I have helped countless people overcome back pain, neck pain, postural fatigue, and work-related musculoskeletal issues. I've spent many years showing people how to set up their workspace and how to sit properly at their desk, so I know firsthand how poor setups can take a toll on the body. The truth is many people aren't fully aware of how their sitting posture and working environment may be affecting their health, until their body starts to complain.

Home Office Handbook: Ergonomic Solutions for Back Pain is a practical guide designed to help remote workers, freelancers, entrepreneurs, and anyone with a home workspace create a healthier, more comfortable way of working. Whether you're dealing with existing pain or looking to prevent it altogether, this book offers actionable solutions based on proven ergonomic principles and real-world experience.

Inside you'll find: Guidance on choosing the right chair, desk, and accessories – Advice for improving posture and reducing strain – Simple ways to stay active, even while seated – Insights into saddle seats, standing desks, kneeling chairs, and other innovative solutions – Case studies, quick tips, and "best practice" checklists.

This handbook is meant to be both a reference and a roadmap. My aim is to empower you with information and inspiration, so you can feel more supported and comfortable throughout your workday, wherever your office may be.

Welcome to a more sustainable way of working.

Dr. Susan Jameson, Chiropractor

Chapter 1

The New Work Landscape

Trend to Remote and Hybrid Work

Work has changed more in the last decade than in the previous half-century. Millions of people now work remotely or in hybrid arrangements, trading commutes for kitchen desks and corporate cubicles for home offices. This flexibility has many rewards — but it also reshapes how our bodies function each day. Without the built-in movement and ergonomic setup of traditional workplaces, back pain has quietly become the new work-from-home epidemic.

Understanding how this shift affects your spine, muscles, and daily habits is the first step toward preventing long-term pain.

The Remote Work Revolution

The COVID-19 pandemic accelerated what was already underway: the digital transformation of work. Overnight, companies adopted remote systems, and workers discovered the comfort — and pitfalls — of home offices. Even post-pandemic, flexibility remains the norm. According to **Owl Labs**, 16 percent of companies worldwide are now fully remote, and nearly two-thirds of workers aged 22 to 65 work from home at least occasionally. [1]

This new reality offers freedom and focus, yet it also removes the physical boundaries that once reminded us to move, stretch, and rest.

How We Adapt to Remote Work

Improvised Workstations

Few homes were designed for full-time office use. Dining chairs, couches, and even beds have become makeshift desks. Poor seating height or monitor alignment forces the spine into awkward curves, straining muscles that were never meant to hold a static position all day.

Less Movement, More Fatigue

In an office, movement happens naturally — walking to a meeting, chatting at a colleague's desk, stepping out for lunch. At home, those micro-breaks vanish. Hours can pass without standing, tightening hip flexors and weakening postural muscles. The result? Stiffness, sluggishness, and a creeping sense of fatigue that drains focus as much as it does comfort.

Blurred Boundaries

Home and work now share the same walls. Many people work longer hours without noticing, rarely pausing to stretch or rest their eyes. Over time, this continuous strain contributes not only to back and neck pain but also to headaches, irritability, and burnout.

> As ergonomics specialist **Dr Samantha Chen** reminds us: "The future of work is flexible — but flexibility demands that we take responsibility for our physical well-being." [2]

How Employers Can Help

Forward-thinking organizations recognise that supporting remote health is an investment in productivity.

Ergonomic Support: Offering stipends or approved checklists for chairs, standing-desk converters, and external keyboards reduces injury risk and absenteeism.

Movement Culture: Encouraging micro-breaks or "walk-and-talk" meetings keeps energy up and tension down.

Wellness Resources: Virtual yoga or stretch sessions, online ergonomic assessments, and mental-health support maintain morale and physical resilience.

Social Connection: Regular virtual coffee breaks or team challenges offset the isolation that often comes with remote work.

Case Studies in Action

Orion Tech's Hybrid Wellness Program

When Orion Tech shifted to hybrid work, engagement dropped and stress soared. The company responded with "Wellness Wednesdays," daily gratitude chats on Slack, and small wellness budgets for managers to tailor support. Within six months, employee engagement rose 35 percent. [3] The lesson: wellbeing initiatives must include social, emotional, and managerial elements — not just physical ergonomics.

Google's Dynamic Workspaces

Google's offices model ergonomic innovation: sit-stand desks, balance-ball seating, treadmill workstations, even "nap pods" for restorative breaks. These initiatives have lowered absenteeism from back pain and boosted creative collaboration. The takeaway for home workers: movement variety isn't a luxury — it's essential fuel for both body and mind.

The Future of Healthy Work

Technology will continue to evolve — AI-driven posture sensors, adaptive furniture, and smarter wellness tracking — but no device can replace the fundamentals: balanced posture, daily movement, and mindful rest. The goal is not perfection but awareness — listening to your body's signals and adjusting before discomfort becomes injury.

Your Next Step

Creating a back-friendly workspace takes experimentation. Adjust your chair height today; schedule short stretch breaks tomorrow. Every small habit compounds into long-term comfort. The more consistently you align and move, the more your back will thank you — with less pain, more energy, and sharper focus.

Looking Ahead

Now that you understand how modern work patterns challenge spinal health, let's explore **how your back actually works** — its structure, the effects of sitting, and the practical habits that keep it strong.

Chapter 2

Taking Care of Your Back

Why Back Health Matters

Back pain is now one of the world's most common health problems. The **World Health Organization** reports that low back pain is the *leading cause of disability globally*, affecting more than 540 million people at any time. Modern lifestyles — prolonged sitting, limited movement, and poor posture — are major culprits. For younger adults, digital work habits have made spinal strain almost inevitable. The economic cost runs into billions each year through lost productivity and treatment.

Caring for your back isn't just about comfort; it's an essential part of protecting your long-term mobility, mood, and quality of life.

Understanding Your Spine

Your spine is a masterpiece of design — flexible yet strong. It contains 33 vertebrae cushioned by discs that act as shock absorbers. Muscles, ligaments, and tendons support the spine.

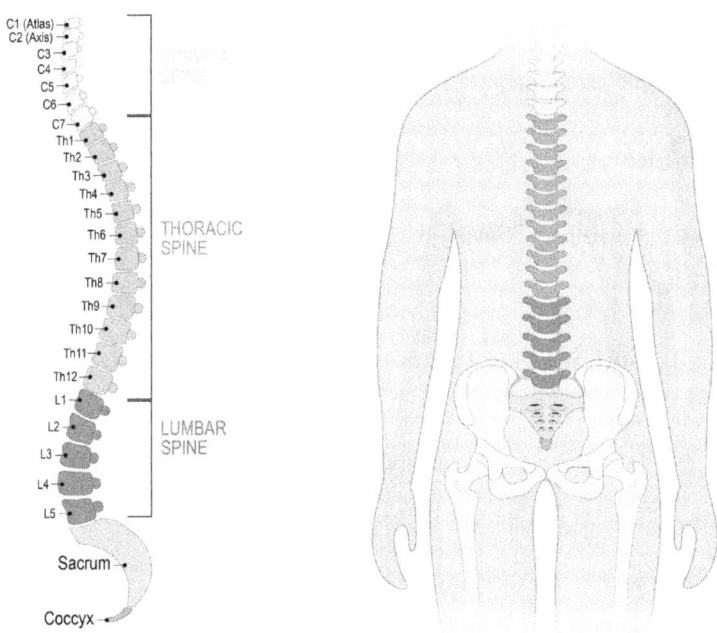

Figure 1 - Diagram of spine showing each area with numbered vertebrae

Cervical (neck): 7 vertebrae

Thoracic (upper back): 12 vertebrae

Lumbar (lower back): 5 vertebrae

Sacrum & Coccyx: fused bones forming your pelvic base

The Risks of Prolonged Sitting

Our spines are built for movement, not for hours of static sitting. When you stay seated too long:

Disc Pressure Rises: Sitting can increase spinal disc pressure by 40 percent compared with standing.

Joints Compress: Reduced movement accelerates arthritic wear, leading to degenerative osteoarthritis in the spine.

Core Weakens: Inactive muscles provide less support.

Circulation Slows: Blood stagnates in the legs, causing swelling and fatigue.

Spine Misaligns: Slouching rounds the shoulders and strains the neck. Think of the spine like a living hinge — it thrives on gentle motion. Without it, stiffness and degeneration will result.

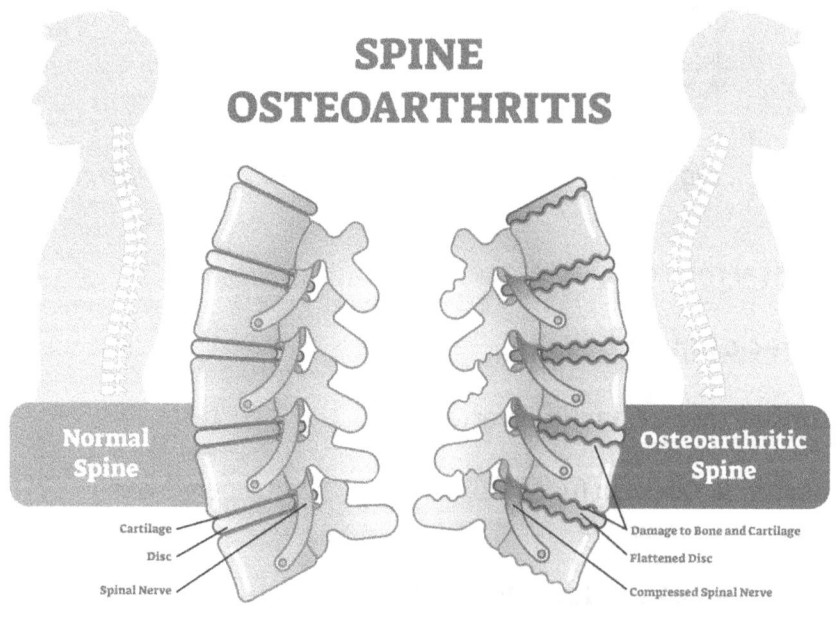

Figure 2 - Diagram of spinal joint osteoarthritis and disc degeneration

Protecting Your Back Daily

A few consistent habits make a powerful difference:

Move Frequently. Stand or stretch every 20 minutes. Use the "20-20-20 rule" — every 20 minutes, move for 20 seconds.

Maintain Neutral Posture. Keep ears, shoulders, and hips aligned when sitting.

Strengthen Your Core. Your abdominal and back muscles act as natural braces for the spine.

Stay Active Outside Work. Walking, swimming, or gentle cycling keeps the body supple and strong.

Smart Exercise for Spine Support

Core Strength

Plank: Forearms on floor, body straight, core engaged — hold 30–60 seconds.

Bird-Dog: From hands and knees, extend opposite arm and leg, pause, then switch.

Dead Bug: Lying on your back, lower opposite arm and leg while keeping your spine flat.

Low-Impact Cardio

Choose movement that's kind to your spine: walking, swimming, cycling, or mini-trampoline (rebounder) sessions. Swimming is ideal because water supports your weight while engaging multiple muscle groups.

Yoga & Pilates

These build flexibility, strength, and body awareness. Try gentle poses like **Cat-Cow**, **Child's Pose**, and **Downward Dog**, or Pilates exercises such as the **Hundred** and **Roll-Up** to strengthen your core with controlled breathing.

Strength Training

When done correctly, squats, deadlifts, and rows fortify the muscles that protect your spine. Start with light resistance, focus on form, and progress gradually — or work with a qualified trainer to avoid injury.

Tip: If you already experience pain, consult a healthcare professional before beginning new exercises.

Nutrition for Spinal Health

A strong back begins with proper fuel.

Healthy Weight: Extra kilos mean extra load on your spine. Choose balanced meals with fruits, vegetables, whole grains, and lean protein.

Hydration: Spinal discs are about 70–80 percent water. Drink roughly 8 glasses daily.

Anti-Inflammatory Foods: Omega-3 sources like salmon, walnuts, and flaxseed help ease inflammation.

Calcium & Vitamin D: Support bone density through leafy greens, dairy, or fortified alternatives, plus moderate sun exposure.

Limit Processed Foods: Reduce sugar and trans-fats that promote inflammation.

Managing Stress to Protect Your Back

Stress tightens muscles — especially across the shoulders and lower back — and amplifies pain perception.

Try simple stress-relief techniques:

Mindfulness Meditation – a few minutes of quiet breathing improves awareness and reduces tension.

Deep Breathing (4-7-8 method): Inhale 4 seconds, hold 7, exhale 8.

Progressive Muscle Relaxation: Tense then relax each body region from toes up.

Sleep Routine: Aim for 7–9 hours nightly; recovery happens during rest.

Stay Connected: Positive social contact lowers cortisol and lifts mood.

When to Seek Professional Help

Contact a health professional if you experience:

Pain lasting more than two weeks

Numbness or tingling in the legs

Pain radiating below the knee

Difficulty controlling bladder or bowel

Pain with fever or unexplained weight loss

Early care prevents minor issues becoming major problems.

The Long-Term Payoff

Back care is a lifelong investment. Every posture correction, stretch, and mindful break reduces your future pain risk. Your spine supports you in everything you do — give it the attention it deserves.

Chapter Summary – 11 Keys to Back Care and Pain Prevention

Create an **ergonomic workspace** with lumbar support and correct screen height.

Take **movement breaks** at least every 20 minutes.

Strengthen your core using safe body-weight exercises.

Engage in **low-impact cardio** such as walking or swimming.

Practice **Yoga or Pilates** to improve flexibility and alignment.

Use **strength training** with proper form and gradual progression.

Maintain a healthy weight with balanced nutrition.

Stay hydrated to protect your spinal discs.

Eat **anti-inflammatory foods** rich in omega-3 fats.

Manage stress through mindfulness, relaxation, and sleep.

Seek professional help when pain persists or new symptoms arise.

Looking Ahead

Now that you understand how to maintain a healthy spine, Chapter 3 will explore **ergonomic workspace design** — how to position your chair, desk, and screen to create a truly back-friendly home office.

Chapter 3

HOME OFFICE ERGONOMICS

The Modern Home Office Challenge

Working from home has redefined what "the office" looks like. Dining tables became desks, kitchen stools became chairs, and laptops replaced monitors. While this flexibility is liberating, it also introduces a hidden risk — poor ergonomics.

A 2021 study by the **American Chiropractic Association** found that **92 percent** of chiropractors reported more patients with back, neck, and shoulder pain after the shift to remote work. [4] This surge highlights one crucial truth: comfort doesn't happen by accident — it must be designed.

The Foundation of Good Ergonomics

Ergonomics is the science of fitting your environment to your body — not the other way around. A properly designed workspace prevents strain, boosts focus, and keeps you feeling energetic throughout the day.

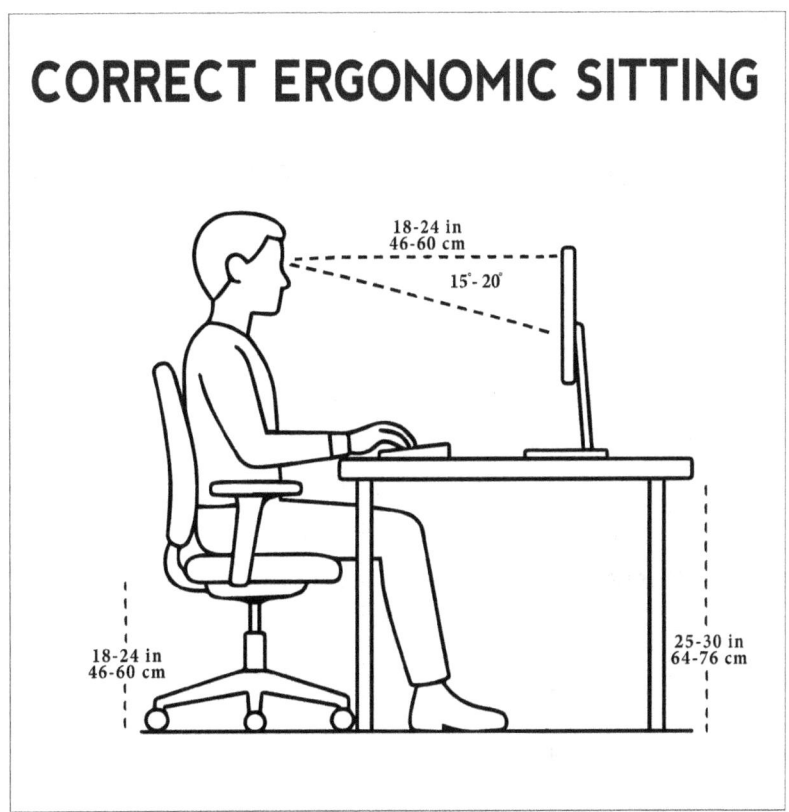

Figure 3 - Correct seated posture

Note – top of monitor at eye level with 15 – 20-degree line of vision to screen

Relaxed arm position, wrists flat

Back supported, feet flat on floor

Key alignment checkpoints include:

Head and neck: balanced over the shoulders, avoiding forward lean.

Shoulders: relaxed, not elevated or rounded.

Elbows: close to the body and bent roughly 90 degrees.

Wrists and hands: straight, not extended upward or downward.

Hips and knees: at or slightly above 90 degrees when sitting.

Feet: flat on the floor or supported by a footrest.

At its core, good ergonomics means maintaining **neutral posture** — ears over shoulders, shoulders over hips, elbows bent at 90 degrees, and wrists straight. Everything in your setup — chair, desk, screen, lighting — should support this alignment.

Creating Your Ergonomic Home Office

Chair – Your Foundation

Your chair supports more than your back; it supports your entire workday. Choose one that offers **lumbar support**, adjustable height, armrests, and a cushioned, breathable seat. Your feet should rest flat on the floor, knees level with or slightly below hips, and your lower back comfortably supported.

If your current chair lacks support, add a **lumbar cushion or a rolled up towel,** and a posture wedge (Chapter 20). These small additions can transform a basic chair into an ergonomic one.

Desk – The Anchor of Alignment

Set your desk so your **elbows rest at 90 degrees** when typing. If it's too high, raise your chair and use a footrest (Chapter 18). If too low, elevate your monitor or laptop with a stand or stack of books.

For adaptable workstyles, consider a **sit-stand desk** (Chapter 5) to vary posture and reduce sitting fatigue.

Monitor – Your Line of Sight

Place the screen directly in front of you, about an arm's length away. The top of the monitor should be at or slightly below eye level, tilting 10–20° backward to reduce glare and neck strain. If you use a laptop, add an **external keyboard and mouse** for proper alignment.

Keyboard and Mouse

Keep wrists straight and elbows close to your body. Move the mouse with your whole arm rather than your wrist to avoid overuse strain. An **ergonomic keyboard** and **vertical mouse** (Chapter 13) can further support neutral wrist position.

Lighting and Environment

Good lighting protects your eyes and supports concentration. Use natural light when possible, balanced with ambient and task lighting. Position screens **perpendicular to windows** to prevent glare.

> As **Dr Mariana Figueiro** from the Light and Health Research Center notes: "Light affects our mood, productivity, and health. In a home office, getting the lighting right is as important as choosing the right chair."

Accessories That Elevate Your Setup

Small accessories can fine-tune comfort and alignment. Consider:

Footrest (Chapter 18) – reduces leg strain when feet don't reach the floor.

Document holder (Chapter 15) – keeps reference material at eye level.

Headset (Chapter 16) – prevents neck twist during calls.

Keyboard tray (Chapter 12) – for optimal typing height.

Lumbar cushion (Chapter 22) and **posture wedge** (Chapter 20) – improve spinal alignment.

Wobble cushion (Chapter 21) – encourages active sitting.

Making Small Spaces Work

Even a compact home office can be ergonomic. Focus on essentials: supportive chair, correct screen height, and keyboard position. Try space-saving options like wall-mounted desks, foldable furniture, or shelving units above your workspace.

Ergonomics isn't about having more space — it's about using the space you have wisely.

Cost-Friendly Comfort

Ergonomics doesn't require expensive equipment. If a full office chair isn't in the budget, enhance what you already have:

Add seat padding (a sheepskin works well).

Use a lumbar cushion or rolled towel.

Employ a footrest or stack of books to reduce pressure.

Elevate your screen with a simple stand or box.

Thoughtful adjustments often make a greater difference than high-price gear.

Healthy Work Habits

A perfect setup is only half the equation. Your body still needs movement, rest, and hydration.

Move often: Follow the 20-20-20 rule — every 20 minutes, look at something 20 feet away for 20 seconds and stand to stretch.

Hydrate: Keep a water bottle on your desk to maintain spinal disc hydration and alertness.

Create boundaries: Define a workspace you can "leave" at day's end to signal mental rest. Simple rituals — shutting your laptop, tidying your desk, stepping outside — help your mind shift from work to recovery.

The Role of Movement

Static posture—whether sitting or standing—causes muscular fatigue and reduced circulation. Micro-movements throughout the day, such as shifting weight, stretching, and standing briefly, help prevent stiffness and discomfort.

Encourage natural movement by:

Adjusting posture every 30–40 minutes.

Standing briefly during phone calls.

Using reminder software or wearable alerts for posture resets.

Regular movement not only maintains spinal flexibility but also enhances energy and concentration.

Accessory Setup and Reach Zones

Frequently used items such as the phone, notebook, or headset should sit within easy reach to minimize twisting and leaning. Arrange the workspace in three zones:

Primary zone: keyboard and mouse.

Secondary zone: frequently accessed items (phone, notepad).

Reference zone: less-used materials or décor.

This simple spatial logic maintains efficiency and protects the spine from repetitive strain.

Temperature, Airflow, and Visual Environment

A comfortable environment reduces muscle tension and fatigue. Maintain room temperature between 20–24 °C (68–75 °F) and ensure good airflow without direct drafts. Natural light exposure supports alertness and circadian rhythm regulation.

Soothing visual elements—plants, gentle colors, or framed images—promote calm focus and can subtly remind the body to breathe and move.

Checkpoints for a Balanced Setup

Sit with back supported and shoulders relaxed.

Keep monitor centered and at eye height.

Maintain elbows near the body at 90°.

Adjust chair height for even hip and knee angles.

Keep feet grounded or supported.

Ensure adequate lighting and limit glare.

Move or stretch at least once every 30–45 minutes.

Prioritize self-care: Stretch, breathe deeply, and sleep well. Physical and mental health are inseparable from postural health.

Common Ergonomic Mistakes

Avoid these frequent pitfalls:

Working from beds or sofas.

Ignoring screen height.

Poor lighting or glare.

Skimping on chair support.

Forgetting movement breaks.

Awareness is the first step toward correction.

The Long-Term Payoff

An ergonomic workspace is an investment in your health, productivity, and well-being. When you support your body properly, you gain energy and focus instead of fatigue and pain. Your workspace should work for you — not against you.

***

Chapter Quick Summary: 15 Keys to Creating an Ergonomic Home Office

Invest in an adjustable chair with lumbar support.

Set desk height for 90° elbow angle.

Position monitor at arm's length and eye level.

Use external keyboard and mouse for laptop work.

Ensure balanced lighting to reduce eye strain.

Add supportive accessories (posture wedge, wobble cushion, footrest).

Follow the 20-20-20 rule for breaks.

Move and stretch every hour.

Keep workspace organized and clutter-free.

Maintain good posture with lumbar support.

Stay hydrated throughout the day.

Alternate between sitting and standing (see Chapter 5).

Adjust your position regularly to avoid stiffness.

Avoid beds and couches for extended work.

Create clear work-life boundaries.

Looking Ahead

With your overall workspace now ergonomically aligned, it's time to focus on the single most important element of that setup — your chair. In the next chapter, we'll explore how choosing and adjusting the right ergonomic chair can make all the difference to your posture, comfort, and long-term spinal health.

Chapter 4

Ergonomic Chairs – The Heart Of Your Setup

Why Your Chair Matters

Your chair is the most critical piece of ergonomic equipment you'll own. We spend up to a third of our lives sitting, and the wrong chair can quietly contribute to stiffness, fatigue, and long-term spinal stress. A well-designed ergonomic chair does far more than provide comfort — it supports **neutral posture**, encourages subtle movement, and allows you to adjust the seat to fit *you*, not the other way around.

The Science of Seating Support

Prolonged sitting can lead to weakened core support muscles, tight hip flexors, rounded shoulders and upper back and forward head posture.

Good seating helps maintain the spine's natural curves and upright posture, while evenly distributing body weight. When your pelvis is supported correctly, the lumbar curve stabilizes, reducing pressure on discs, joints and surrounding muscles. The upper body can then realign to a more optimal posture.

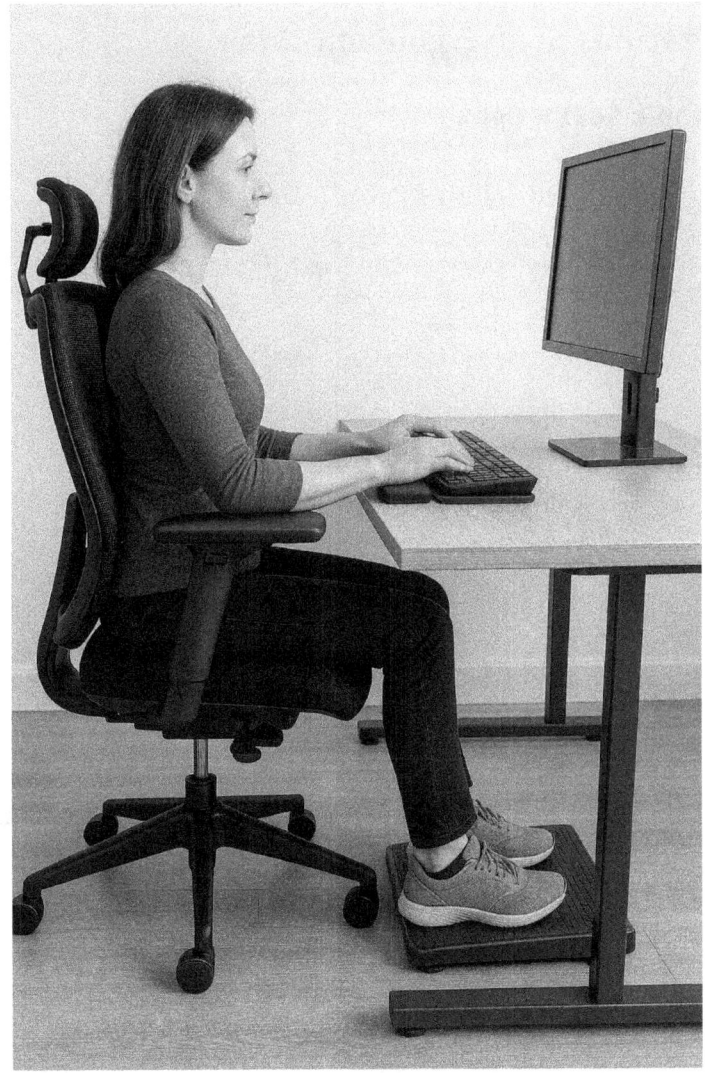

Figure 4 - Correct seated posture at a computer workstation.

Correct sitting posture: note the upright back supported by the chair, feet on a footrest, elbows at approximately 90 degrees, and top of the monitor at eye level.

Key Features of an Ergonomic Chair

Adjustable Seat Height

Knees level with or slightly below hips.

Feet flat on the floor or on a **footrest** (Chapter 18).

Lumbar Support

The small of your back should contact the chair's curve at waist height.

Some ergonomic chairs have adjustable lumbar support.

For extra comfort, add a **lumbar cushion** if needed (Chapter 22).

Seat Depth and Width

Leave a 2–3 cm gap between the seat edge and back of the knees.

Shorter users may need a sliding seat pan or small-frame model.

Backrest Recline, Tilt and Tension control

A slight recline (100–110°) reduces disc pressure.

Dynamic tilt mechanisms help reduce lumbar compression and encourage micro-movements that keep spinal muscles active.

Armrests

Height-adjustable to keep shoulders relaxed.

Drop-away or pivoting designs work best with sit-stand desks (Chapter 5).

Seat Material and Breathability

Mesh backs improve airflow.

High-density foam cushions distribute pressure evenly.

Mobility and Stability

Five-point base for balance.

Modern ergonomic chairs are built around **adjustability** — every person's proportions differ, so flexibility is the true measure of good design.

Setting Up Your Chair Correctly

Adjust the height so your **elbows are level with the desk surface**.

Ensure your **hips are slightly higher than knees**.

Keep your **shoulders relaxed** and **wrists straight**.

Sit back fully against the lumbar support.

Case Study – Autodesk's Seating Redesign

When Autodesk upgraded its offices, employees were encouraged to select adjustable ergonomic chairs and receive professional fitting. After six months:

52% reported less lower-back discomfort.

41% reported improved concentration. The investment paid off in fewer absences and higher morale — proof that supportive seating drives both health and performance.

Emerging Trends in Ergonomic Seating

Smart Chairs: Sensors now track posture and remind users to move.

Eco Designs: Manufacturers use recycled mesh and bio-foam materials.

Hybrid Seating: Chairs that convert to stools or perches support flexible working styles.

Saddle and Kneeling Options: See **Chapters 8 and 9** for posture-enhancing alternatives.

The Long-Term Payoff

A supportive chair protects your spine, reduces fatigue, and keeps your energy consistent throughout the day. Think of it as an investment in decades of comfort and productivity. Combine quality seating with **movement breaks** and **stretching routines** for the best results.

***

Chapter Quick Summary – 11 Keys to Choosing and Using an Ergonomic Chair

Adjustable seat height and depth.

Supportive lumbar curve.

Slight recline for spinal relief.

Armrests at relaxed shoulder level.

Breathable materials.

Stable five-point base.

Correct seat-to-desk height.

Neutral wrist and elbow angles.

Regular movement and micro-breaks.

Supplement with cushions or wedges as needed.

Re-evaluate setup whenever your tasks change.

Looking Ahead

Your chair is now optimized for comfort and alignment — but no matter how supportive it is, static sitting still challenges your spine. Next, in Chapter 5, we explore **standing and sit-stand desks**, the modern tools that bring movement back into the workday.

Chapter 5

Standing Desks: A Game-Changer In Back Care

Why Standing Desks Matter

For decades, office work meant long hours of sitting — a posture now linked to back pain, fatigue, and metabolic issues. Standing desks emerged as a powerful alternative, encouraging more movement and offering a way to break the cycle of prolonged sitting. These desks, available as fixed-height or adjustable models, help restore the body's natural rhythm of motion and alignment.

Standing desks aren't about replacing sitting entirely. They're about **bringing balance back** to your day by promoting posture variation, improved circulation, and greater comfort.

Making the Transition

Switching to a standing desk should be gradual. Begin with **15–30 minutes per hour** of standing and increase slowly as your body adapts. Early fatigue is normal — muscles simply need time to strengthen.

When standing:

Keep your screen **at eye level**.

Position your keyboard and mouse so elbows rest at **90 degrees**. Using a keyboard tray (Chapter 13) under the desktop lowers the keyboard height.

Distribute your weight evenly on both feet.

Use an **anti-fatigue mat** for cushioning. It promotes gentle movement in the feet and legs, improving comfort and reducing pressure.

Alternate positions every **30–60 minutes**.

Key Insight: The goal isn't to stand all day — it's to move more and sit less.

Sit-Stand Desks: Flexibility for Modern Work

A sit-stand desk (also called an adjustable-height desk) lets you switch between sitting and standing at the touch of a button or lever. This adaptability supports spinal health and energy balance.

Interesting Fact: Researchers at the **University of Leicester** found that standing just **three extra hours a day** can burn up to

30 000 extra calories per year — roughly equivalent to running 10 marathons. [7]

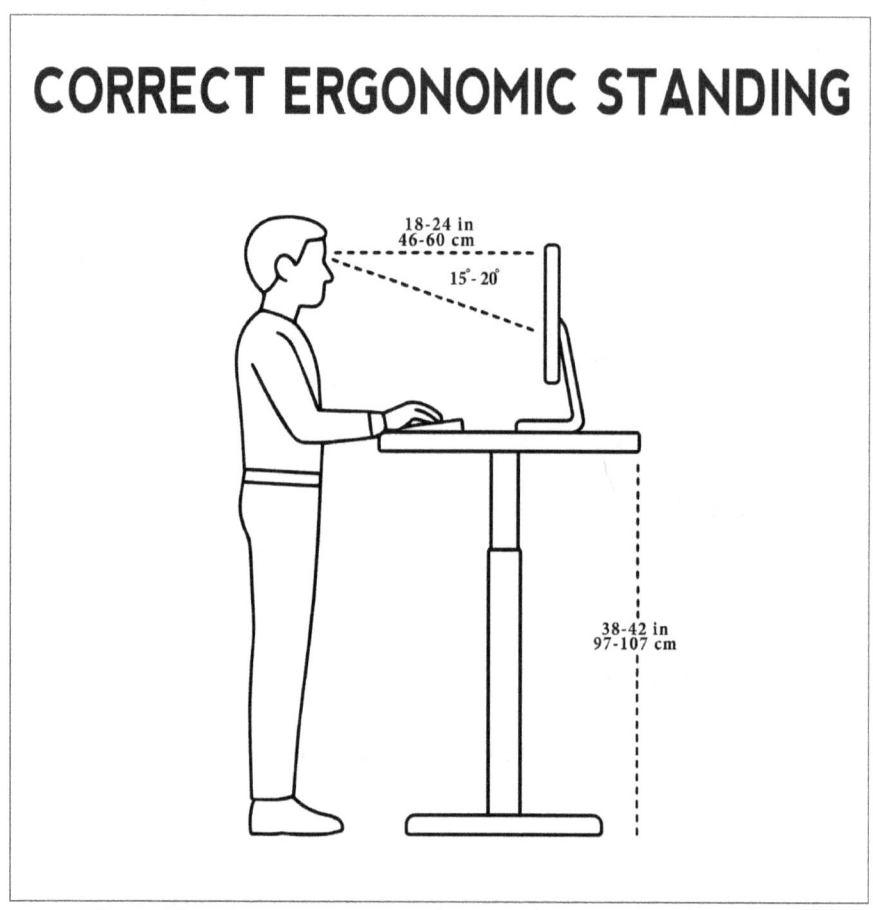

Figure 5 – Correct ergonomic posture at a standing desk

Evidence for Sit-Stand Success

Scientific research strongly supports the benefits of sit-stand work. A **2021 study in the *Journal of Occupational Health*** reported that workers alternating every 30 minutes between sitting and standing experienced a **32 percent reduction in lower-back pain** and higher energy levels. [8]

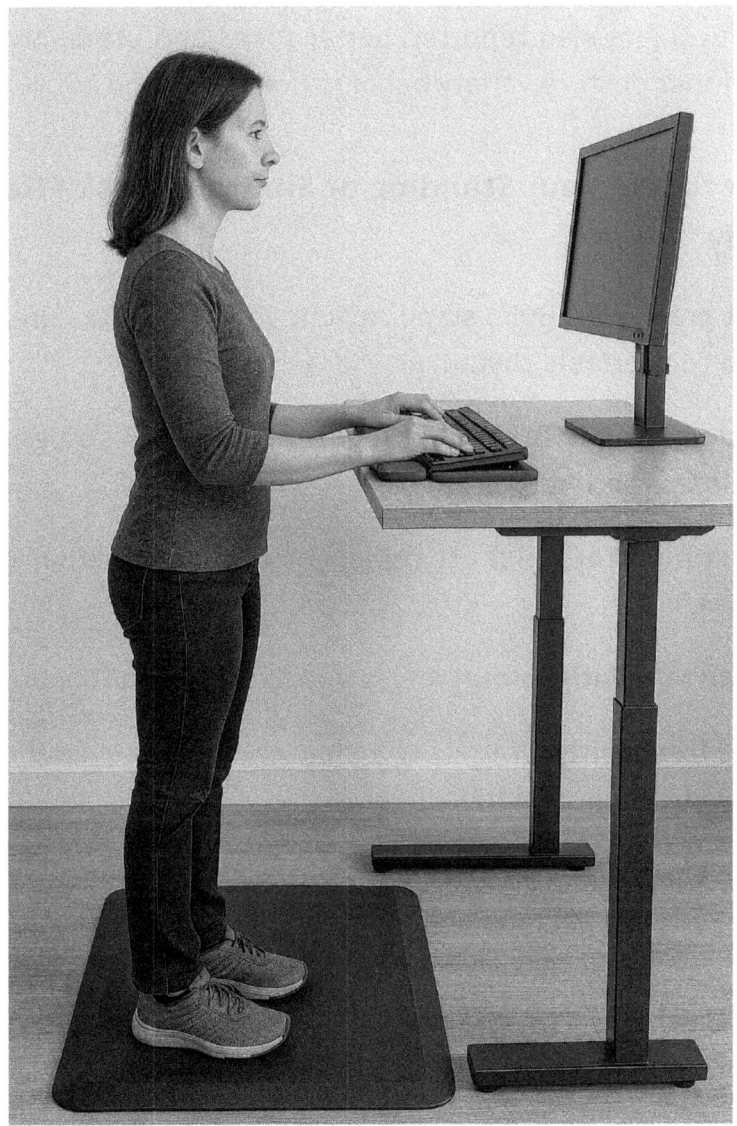

Figure 6 - Standing desk posture. Note use of fatigue mat, top of monitor at eye level with 15 to 20 degree line of vision to screen, upright posture, relaxed arms, wrists flat.

Another investigation in the *Journal of Occupational and Environmental Medicine* showed a **54 percent drop in upper-back and neck pain** after only four weeks of sit-stand desk use.[9] Participants also reported better focus and productivity — proof that posture variety benefits both body and mind.

How to Use Your Standing or Sit-Stand Desk Effectively

Start gradually. Build standing time in short blocks until you find a comfortable rhythm.

Set desk height at elbow level. Keep wrists straight and shoulders relaxed.

Adjust monitor height to remain at eye level whether sitting or standing.

Use an anti-fatigue mat for leg and foot comfort (Chapter 19).

Move frequently. Walk or stretch every hour — even the best desk can't replace motion.

Wear supportive shoes. Flat, cushioned footwear minimizes strain during long standing periods.

The Benefits at a Glance

Less Back Pain: Sit-stand use reduces pressure on spinal discs.

Improved Posture: Standing naturally activates core muscles, countering slouching habits.

More Energy & Focus: Dynamic posture boosts blood flow and alertness.

Lower Disease Risk: Less sedentary time supports cardiovascular and metabolic health.

Increased Calorie Burn: Small daily gains add up over time.

Potential Drawbacks

Like any new routine, sit-stand use has an adjustment period.

Initial soreness: Muscles may fatigue before they strengthen.

Cost and space: High-quality desks require investment and room to operate.

Overuse: Standing too long without variation can also cause strain — balance is key.

The Bottom Line

Standing and sit-stand desks represent one of the most practical ergonomic advances of modern work. When used correctly, they encourage movement, support spinal health, and enhance overall vitality.

Integrate your desk into a **holistic posture plan** — include regular stretching, exercise, and good nutrition. These combined habits will protect your back, energize your body, and keep your workday pain-free.

Chapter Quick Summary – 18 Keys to Using Standing and Sit-Stand Desks

Start with short standing intervals (15–30 min).

Aim for a 1 : 1 – 1 : 3 standing-to-sitting ratio.

Keep desk height at elbow level.

Monitor at eye level, arm's length away.

Use an anti-fatigue mat for comfort.

Maintain neutral spine alignment.

Balance weight evenly on both feet.

Move and stretch hourly.

Adjust if discomfort arises.

Stay hydrated.

Wear supportive shoes.

Use reminders to change positions.

Increase standing time gradually.

Combine desk use with walking or stretching.

Set ergonomics correctly for both positions.

Add a keyboard tray for wrist support.

Re-set monitor height when switching posture.

Incorporate daily stretching for flexibility.

Looking Ahead

Now that you've mastered standing and sit-stand techniques, let's explore the next level of dynamic ergonomics — **active sitting**. In Chapter 6, you'll learn how movement-based seating options, like saddle stools and wobble cushions, keep your body engaged even while seated.

Chapter 6

ACTIVE SITTING SOLUTIONS AND DYNAMIC POSTURE

The Problem with Static Sitting

Even with the best ergonomic chair, long hours of stillness can take a toll. Human bodies are built to move — muscles, joints, and even intervertebral discs rely on regular motion to stay healthy. Static postures, whether sitting or standing, can restrict circulation, weaken muscles, and lead to fatigue or pain.

Active sitting offers a practical solution. By encouraging subtle movement throughout the day, it keeps the body engaged, stimulates core muscles, and helps maintain spinal alignment.

What Is Active Sitting?

Active sitting (also called *dynamic sitting*) involves using seating that allows and encourages small, controlled movements. This motion keeps your stabilizing muscles active and prevents stiffness caused by static posture. Instead of locking your body into one position, active seating promotes gentle balance adjustments that mimic the body's natural movement patterns.

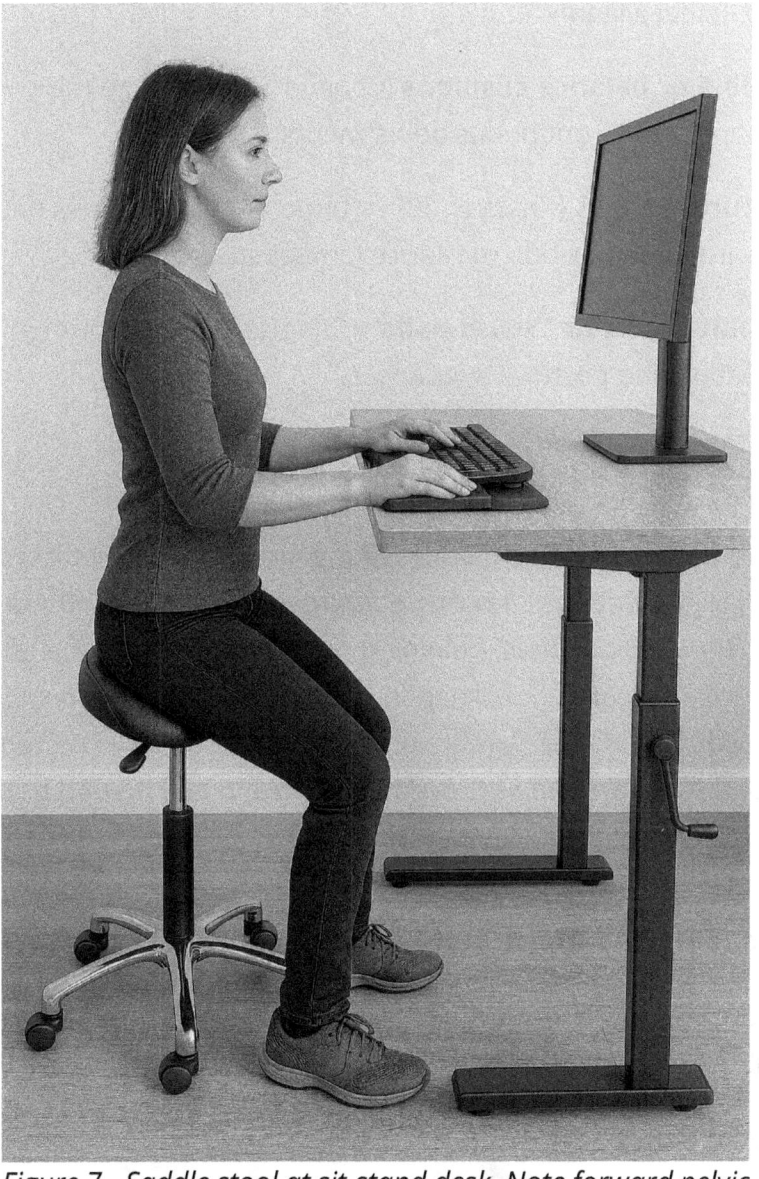

Figure 7 - Saddle stool at sit-stand desk. Note forward pelvic tilt, lumbar curve and upright posture

Common examples of active sitting include:

Saddle stools (Chapter 8) – promote an open hip angle and upright spinal alignment.

Wobble or balance cushions (Chapter 21) – engage the core by creating small, continuous adjustments.

Posture wedges (Chapter 20) – support the pelvis in a neutral, forward-tilted position to reduce lumbar strain.

Stability balls or "Swiss balls" (Chapter 10) – encourage core activation and postural awareness.

The Science Behind Movement

Movement is a form of medicine for your musculoskeletal system. Even slight changes in posture improve blood flow and nutrient delivery to spinal discs, helping them maintain hydration and resilience. Research published in the *Journal of Occupational Rehabilitation* found that workers using dynamic seating reported less back discomfort and improved concentration compared to those using fixed chairs.[10]

Choosing the Right Active Sitting Option

When selecting a dynamic seating device, consider comfort, adjustability, and how it integrates into your workspace.

Saddle Stools

Saddle stools mimic the posture of horseback riding — knees below hips, spine naturally aligned, and pelvis slightly forward.

This position opens the hip angle, reduces lumbar pressure, and encourages a balanced, upright spine. Saddle stools pair well with **standing or sit-stand desks** (Chapter 5) and are ideal for short to moderate use throughout the day.

Wobble Cushions and Balance Stools

These options introduce gentle instability, prompting continuous micro-adjustments in your abdominal and back muscles. Over time, they help develop balance, strength, and postural awareness. Start slowly — 15 to 20 minutes at a time — until your muscles adapt.

Posture Wedges and Seat Cushions

These create a forward pelvic tilt that helps maintain the spine's natural S-curve. A small angle (10–15°) is enough to relieve lower-back tension and promote upright posture. Pair posture wedges with an **ergonomic chair** (Chapter 4) or **sit-stand desk** (Chapter 5) for best results.

Stability Balls

Sitting on a stability ball can engage the core and improve balance, but it's best used occasionally. Extended use without back support may cause fatigue. Consider alternating between your main chair and the ball for short work sessions or stretching breaks.

Integrating Movement into Your Day

Active sitting is most effective when combined with other healthy habits. Here's how to make it part of your daily rhythm:

Alternate positions regularly. Switch between chair, stool, and standing desk throughout the day.

Take movement breaks. Every hour, stand, stretch, or walk for a few minutes.

Use micro-movements. Gentle pelvic tilts or shoulder rolls help maintain circulation.

Engage your core consciously. While sitting, imagine lengthening your spine and drawing your navel slightly inward.

Stay hydrated. Regular water intake encourages you to stand, refill, and move naturally.

Set reminders. Use a timer or posture app to prompt movement if you lose track of time.

The Benefits of Active Sitting

Active sitting can dramatically improve comfort, focus, and overall well-being. Key benefits include:

Enhanced Core Strength: Continuous micro-movements engage abdominal and back muscles.

Reduced Back Pain: Frequent posture changes minimize spinal stress.

Improved Circulation: Dynamic posture boosts oxygen flow and prevents stiffness.

Better Focus and Energy: Small movements stimulate alertness and reduce fatigue.

Encouraged Postural Awareness: Movement builds a natural habit of alignment and balance.

> As ergonomist **Dr Mark Benden** from Texas A&M University notes, "The goal of good seating isn't stillness — it's supported motion."

Potential Drawbacks and Tips

Active sitting should feel natural and comfortable, not tiring or unstable.

Start gradually — 10–20 minutes at a time.

Avoid sitting so low that your knees rise above hips.

Combine with **ergonomic chair use** for support during longer tasks.

Maintain posture awareness; movement should enhance, not replace, good alignment.

If you feel discomfort or muscle fatigue, return to a supported chair and stretch. Your endurance will improve with time.

The Bigger Picture

Dynamic posture isn't just about special chairs — it's a mindset. Whether you're sitting, standing, or walking, your goal is variation. Every posture has value when it's part of a balanced movement routine.

The more you move, the better your spine performs. By embracing active sitting, you transform ordinary desk time into a low-intensity workout for your postural health.

***

Chapter Quick Summary – 14 Keys to Active Sitting and Dynamic Posture

Use dynamic seating (saddle stool, wobble cushion, or posture wedge).

Maintain an open hip angle with knees below hips.

Keep your spine tall and core gently engaged.

Begin with short sessions, increasing over time.

Switch between sitting, standing, and moving.

Use a stability ball occasionally to strengthen balance.

Combine active sitting with regular movement breaks.

Avoid static positions for more than an hour.

Adjust seating height for elbow and eye-level alignment.

Hydrate regularly to maintain focus and spinal health.

Practice gentle micro-movements while seated.

Listen to your body and rest if discomfort arises.

Combine with stretching and posture checks (see Chapter 7).

Think "move more, hold less" — variation is vitality.

Looking Ahead

We've now explored how movement, posture variation, and active sitting transform your workspace into a healthier, more dynamic environment. In the next chapter, we'll look at how to troubleshoot common ergonomic challenges and fine-tune your setup.

Chapter 7

Troubleshooting Your Ergonomic Setup

When Comfort Still Feels Out of Reach

Even with an excellent ergonomic setup, small issues can persist. A chair that's too firm, a monitor that's slightly low, or hours without movement can all lead to discomfort. The good news: most problems can be corrected with a few mindful tweaks and consistent habits.

This chapter will help you identify common trouble spots, fine-tune your workspace, and build flexibility into your daily routine so your posture — and productivity — stay strong.

Persistent Back Pain

If your back still aches after improving your setup, look deeper than the chair itself.

Quick fixes to try:

Add a **lumbar cushion** centred at the small of your back.

Sit on a **posture wedge** (Chapter 20) to restore the spine's natural curve, or a **wobble cushion to create more movement** (Chapter 21)

Alternate between **sitting and standing** more often using a sit-stand or standing desk (Chapter 5).

Incorporate **Active Sitting** strategies (Chapter 6).

If pain persists, consult a qualified health professional.

Neck Strain

Neck tension usually stems from poor screen alignment. Ensure the monitor's top edge sits at **eye level**, about **an arm's length** away. If you use dual screens, keep your main display directly in front of you and angle the secondary one toward you. An **adjustable headrest** can help relieve neck muscles; increasing lumbar support also realigns the upper spine to reduce pressure.

Wrist or Forearm Pain

Pain in the wrists or forearms often indicates strain from incorrect keyboard or mouse placement.

Keep wrists **neutral**, not bent up or down.

Use a **wrist rest** or **ergonomic keyboard and mouse** (Chapter 13).

Install a **keyboard tray** (Chapter 12) to keep arms at a relaxed 90-degree angle.

Eye Strain and Fatigue

Digital eyestrain is common in bright or poorly lit spaces.

Position your screen perpendicular to windows to avoid glare.

Balance **natural light** with soft task lighting.

Follow the **20-20-20 rule** — every 20 minutes, look 20 feet away for 20 seconds.

Consider **blue-light-filter glasses** for extended computer use.

Fatigue from Standing

If you're new to a standing desk, early fatigue is normal.

Gradually increase standing periods.

Use an **anti-fatigue mat** (Chapter 19) and **supportive footwear**.

Alternate between sitting, standing, and moving — variety prevents strain.

The "Flex and Flow" Method

To help ergonomics become second nature, use the **Flex and Flow** method — a simple cycle that blends posture awareness with regular movement.

Flex: Adjust your workspace to match your current task — raise or lower the desk, reposition the monitor, or modify your chair.

Flow: Work for 30–60 minutes with steady posture and focused attention.

Move: When the timer rings, stretch, stand, or walk briefly.

Reassess: Before resuming, notice your body. Do you feel tightness, tension, or fatigue? Adjust accordingly.

Repeat: Cycle through this rhythm all day. Small resets keep your muscles active and your concentration sharp.

This routine blends equipment efficiency with body awareness — making ergonomics less about furniture and more about daily mindfulness.

Action Steps for Ergonomic Success

Assess your workspace. Identify areas that cause discomfort.

Invest strategically. A supportive chair and height-adjustable desk are worth the cost.

Fine-tune alignment. Review **monitor and keyboard positions** (Chapters 3 & 4) regularly.

Practice Flex and Flow three to four cycles daily; increase as it becomes habit.

Integrate Active Sitting (Chapter 6) for short sessions.

Record progress — track comfort, focus, and fatigue.

Consult professionals if symptoms persist.

Stay adaptable. Bodies change, and so should work habits.

Cultivating an Ergonomic Mindset

Ergonomics is a lifelong practice, not a one-time setup. Stay tuned to your body, make small daily adjustments, and remain curious about new tools or techniques.

Your healthiest workspace is one that evolves with you — supporting not only your spine, but your energy, focus, and overall well-being.

***

Chapter Quick Summary – 9 Keys for Troubleshooting Your Ergonomic Setup

Evaluate your current setup for problem areas.

Invest in key tools like a quality chair or sit-stand desk.

Add accessories — lumbar support, posture wedge, or wobble cushion — as needed.

Follow workstation alignment rules for screens and keyboards.

Use the **Flex and Flow** method three to four times a day.

Practice **Active Sitting** (Chapter 6) to encourage movement.

Keep a one-month **Companion Journal** to monitor changes.

Seek professional help if pain continues.

Stay adaptable — adjust your environment as your needs evolve.

Looking Ahead

With your workspace fine-tuned and the Flex and Flow method in place, you're ready to explore alternative seating options.

Chapter 8

Saddle Seats: Ergonomic Seating Revolution

The Rise of Active Seating

Originally designed for dentists, **saddle seats** have become a favorite among professionals seeking better posture and relief from back pain. Inspired by horseback riding, their forward-tilted shape promotes an open hip angle and upright spine — a posture that aligns naturally with human anatomy.

Why Saddle Seats Work

Traditional chairs often tilt the pelvis backward, flattening the lumbar curve and increasing disc pressure. In contrast, saddle seats **tilt the pelvis slightly forward**, maintaining spinal alignment and creating a more active sitting position. The result: improved comfort, better circulation, and greater awareness of posture.

Key Benefits

Improved Posture: Hips higher than knees preserve the spine's natural S-curve.

Core Engagement: The seat's balance point keeps abdominal and back muscles active.

Better Circulation: Open hip angles enhance blood flow to legs and feet.

Freedom of Movement: Compact design allows easy mobility around the workspace.

Reduced Internal Pressure: Forward tilt eases compression on internal organs, improving comfort and digestion.

Choosing the Right Saddle Seat

When selecting your saddle stool, consider:

Adjustability: Height and tilt controls let you fine-tune comfort.

Seat Design: Split models reduce pressure on sensitive areas.

Material: Durable, breathable fabric improves comfort for longer use.

Base Stability: A five-wheel base ensures balance and smooth movement.

> Dr James Levine of the Mayo Clinic said it best: "The best posture is the next posture." This philosophy defines the saddle seat — encouraging constant, supported motion throughout the day.

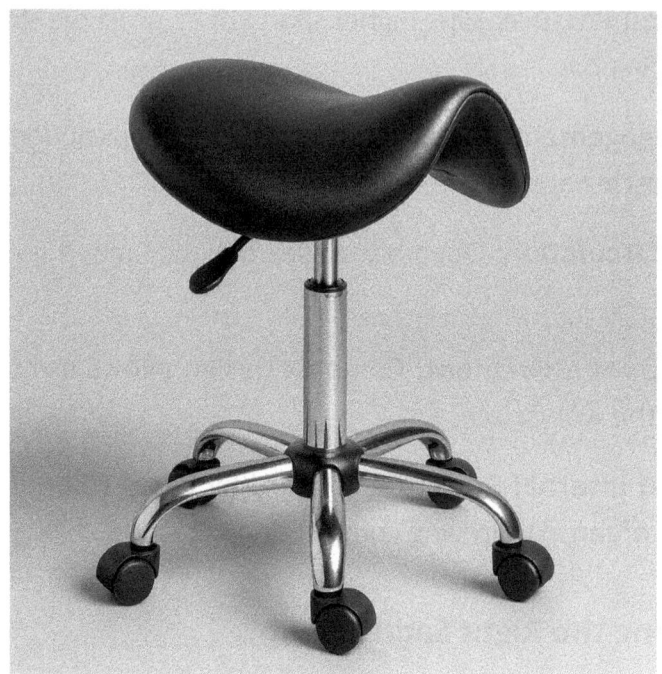

Figure 7 - A saddle stool supports active sitting

Integrating a Saddle Seat

Start Slowly: Begin with 15–30 minutes at a time; increase as your body adapts.

Adjust Stool Height: A saddle stool can be used at normal desk height or raised when used with a **sit-stand desk** (Chapter 6) **for positional variation**

Stay Aware of Posture: Keep the spine tall, shoulders relaxed, feet grounded.

Take Regular Breaks: Stand, stretch, or walk every hour.

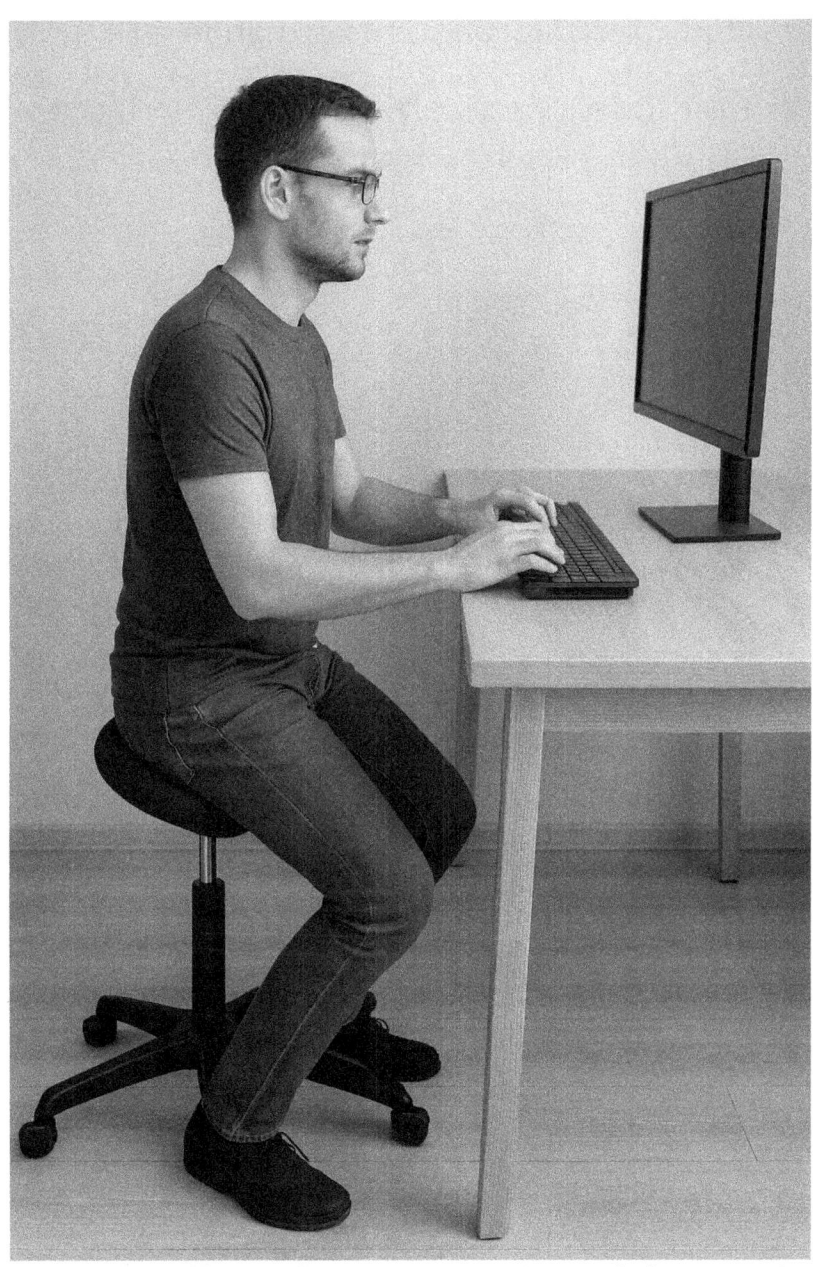
Figure 8 - A saddle stool supports active sitting. It helps maintains the lumbar curve and engages the core support muscles

Case Study: Tech Startup Transformation

A San Francisco tech startup introduced saddle stools to replace traditional chairs. After three months:

70% of employees reported less lower-back pain.

85% noticed improved posture.

60% felt more energetic.

40% reported better focus.

These results illustrate how seating design can transform both comfort and productivity.

The Bigger Picture

Saddle seats are a breakthrough, but they're just one tool in a holistic approach to spinal wellness. Combine them with **Active Sitting** (Chapter 6), movement breaks, and ergonomic workspace design for lasting benefits.

***

Chapter Quick Summary – 13 Keys to Maximizing Saddle Seat Benefits

Begin with 15–30 minutes per session.

Gradually increase duration as muscles adapt.

Adjust desk and monitor height for proper posture.

Maintain a neutral spine and open hip angle.

Take standing breaks every hour.

Pair with a **standing desk** (Chapter 5) for posture variation.

Choose adjustable, breathable designs.

Ensure base stability and smooth-rolling casters.

Try split-seat models for pressure relief.

Engage your core gently throughout the day.

Improve circulation with relaxed leg position.

Use durable materials for comfort and longevity.

Remember: variation is key — alternate with other seats.

Looking Ahead

By now you should be getting the idea of what active sitting is all about. In the next chapter we will explore kneeling chairs, another active sitting device.

Chapter 9

KNEELING CHAIRS TO REDUCE BACK PAIN

A Forward-Leaning Solution

The **kneeling chair** redistributes body weight between the buttocks and shins, tilting the pelvis forward and encouraging the spine's natural curve. Originally introduced in the 1970s, it remains one of the most recognizable alternatives to traditional office seating.

How It Works

By shifting your center of gravity forward, a kneeling chair aligns the head, shoulders, and hips while reducing lumbar disc pressure. The result is a posture that activates the core and encourages dynamic balance — similar in philosophy to **saddle seating** (Chapter 8) but with added support from the knees.

Benefits of Kneeling Chairs

Better Posture: Forward tilt preserves the lumbar curve.

Reduced Back Pain: Relieves lower-back stress by shifting weight forward.

Core Strength: Requires small, continuous balance adjustments.

Improved Circulation: Open hip angles enhance blood flow to legs.

Posture Awareness: keeps you mindful of alignment while working.

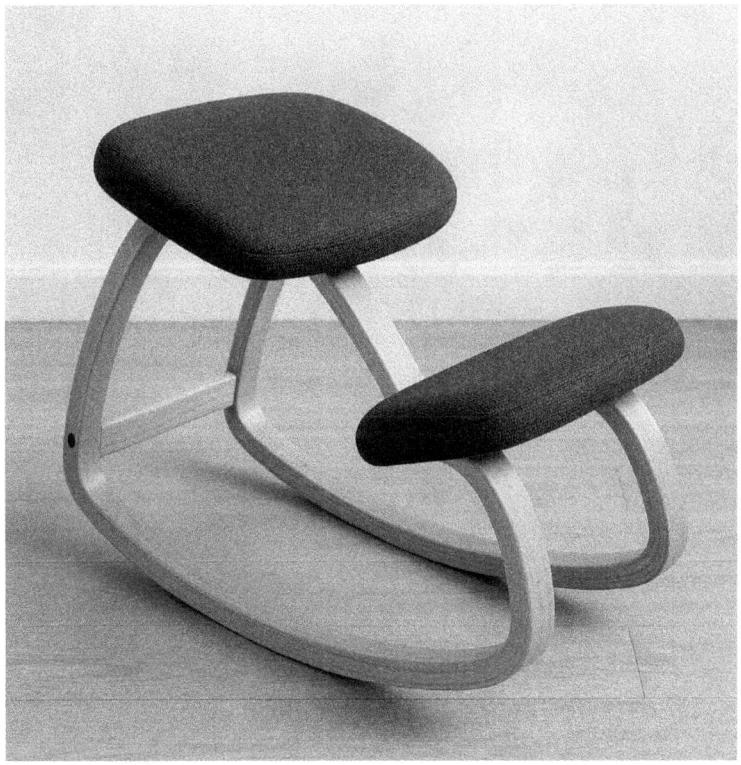

(Figure 10 – Rocker kneeling chairs add dynamic movement and core engagement)

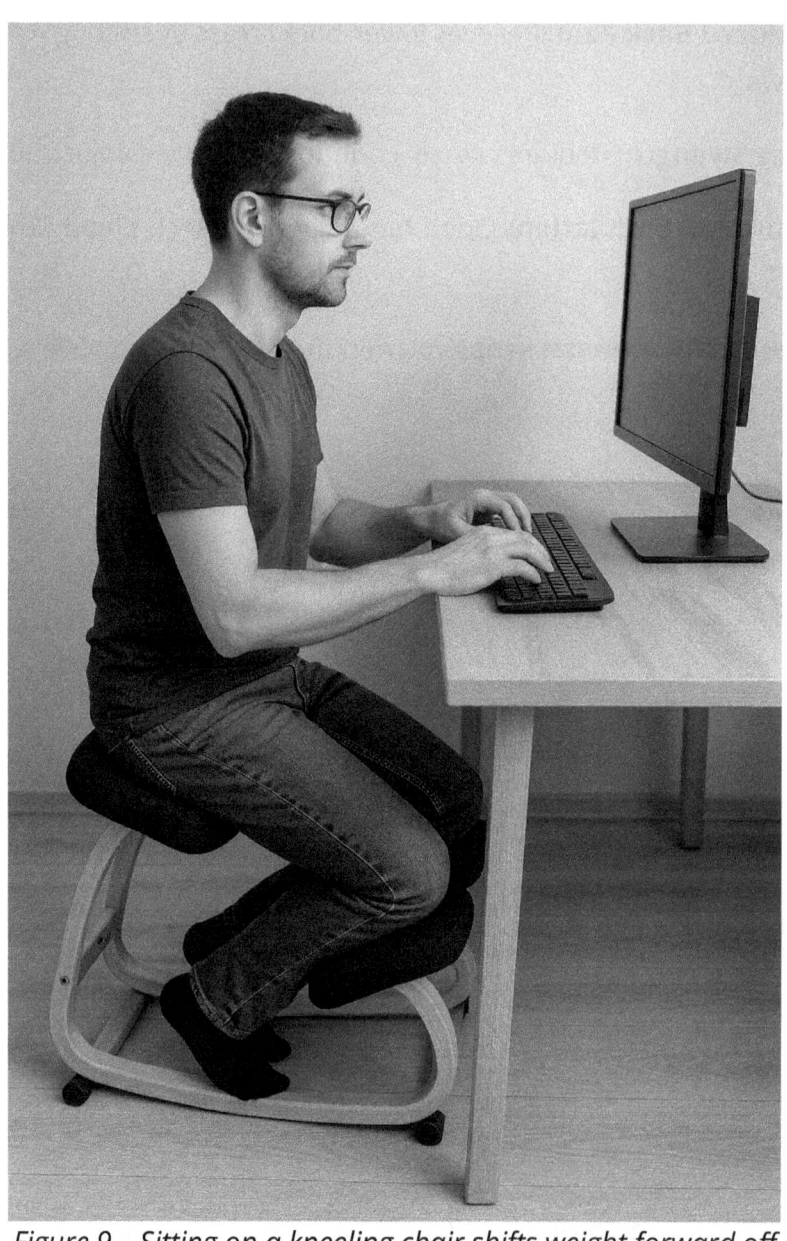

Figure 9 – Sitting on a kneeling chair shifts weight forward off the spine to the legs

Using a Kneeling Chair Safely

Start Gradually: Begin with short sessions (15–30 minutes).

Alternate Seating: Switch between kneeling and regular chairs during the day.

Adjust Your Workspace: Realign your monitor and keyboard.

Balance Weight Evenly: Share weight between buttocks and shins.

Stretch Frequently: Move or stand every 30–60 minutes.

Consultation: If you have knee issues, check suitability with a health provider.

Avoid Overuse: Kneeling chairs aren't suited for all-day sitting.

Contraindication: Don't use a kneeling chair if you have ongoing knee issues.

Special Applications

Musicians, dentists, and creative professionals often use kneeling chairs to maintain posture during precision work.

Newer models include rocking bases for **Active Sitting**, merging movement with spinal alignment.

***

Chapter Quick Summary – 8 Keys for Using Kneeling Chairs

Start slowly and increase usage gradually.

Alternate between kneeling and traditional chairs.

Maintain even weight distribution.

Adjust workspace for new posture.

Keep your spine tall and shoulders relaxed.

Include stretching breaks every hour.

Strengthen your core for long-term comfort.

Use as part of a varied ergonomic routine.

Looking Ahead

In the next chapter, we explore the **stability ball**, a versatile tool that transforms sitting into an active, core-strengthening experience.

Chapter 10

Stability Ball - A Versatile Tool For Back Pain Relief

From Therapy to Office Essential

First used in physical therapy, **stability balls** — also called exercise or Swiss balls — have found a home in modern offices. Their gentle instability keeps the body in motion, promoting balance and strengthening deep core muscles.

Why It Works

Sitting on a stability ball requires continuous micro-adjustments, which:

Activate core stabilizing muscles in the abdomen and back.

Promote upright posture and spinal alignment.

Improve blood circulation through subtle movement.

Stability balls are best used **in short intervals** as part of a movement-friendly routine.

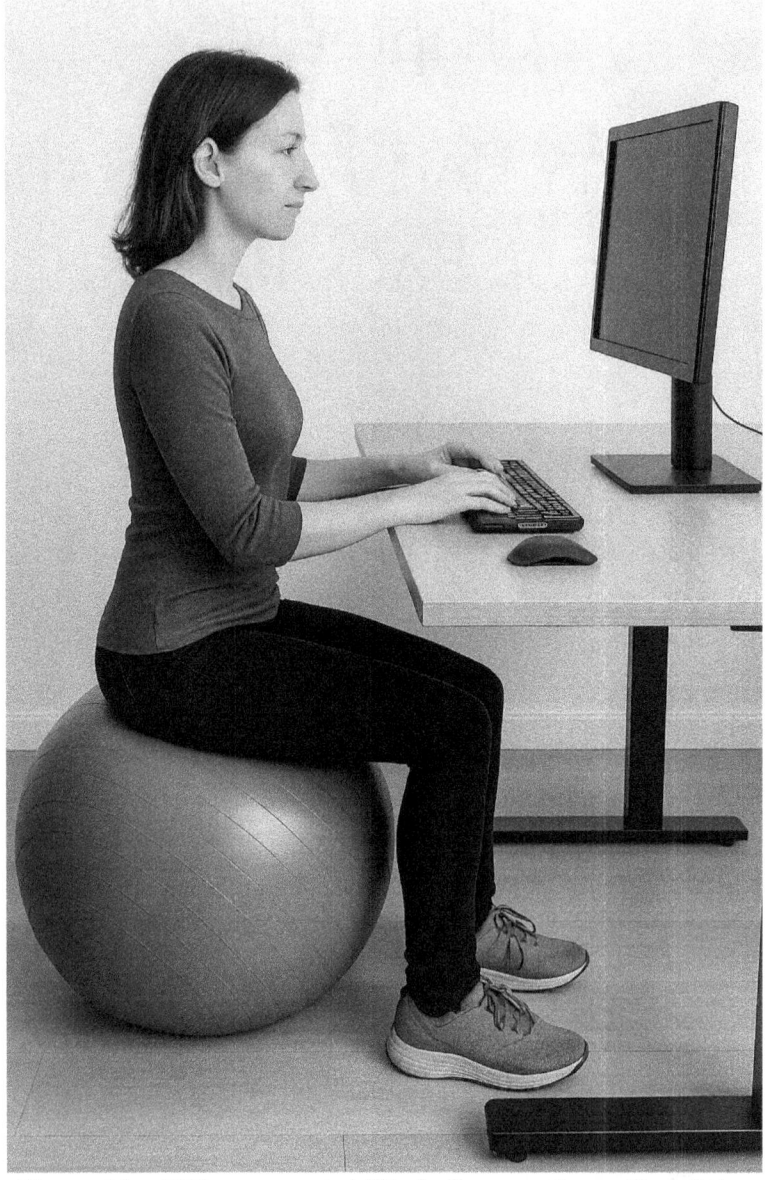

Figure 11 – Sitting on a stability ball promotes active sitting and core engagement

Benefits of Stability Balls

Improved Posture: Encourages neutral spine alignment.

Core Strengthening: Builds endurance in postural muscles.

Increased Circulation: Prevents stiffness and fatigue.

Enhanced Focus: Movement stimulates brain activity and energy.

Variety: Offers a refreshing alternative to static seating.

Potential Drawbacks

While beneficial, stability balls have limitations:

No Back Support: Not ideal for people with existing spinal conditions.

Fatigue: Prolonged sitting can cause muscle soreness.

Stability Concerns: Risk of rolling or imbalance.

Limited Adjustability: Unlike chairs, height and support are fixed.

How to Use a Stability Ball

Start Slowly: Use for 15–30 minutes per session.

Maintain Posture: Keep your spine tall, shoulders relaxed, and feet flat.

Alternate Seating: Mix with a traditional or ergonomic chair.

Add Movement: Try gentle bouncing, pelvic tilts, or seated marches.

Use a Base or Stand: Adds stability for longer sessions.

Take Breaks: Stand and stretch every 30-60 minutes.

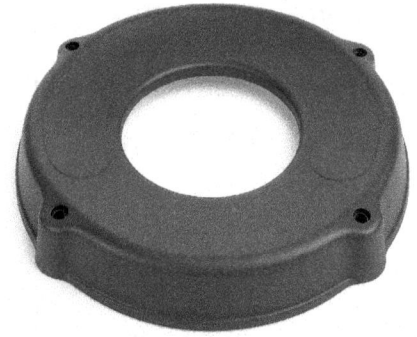

Figure 12 – Stability ball base adds safety and reduces rolling, making it ideal for longer use

Exercises to Enhance Stability Ball Benefits

Incorporating simple exercises while seated on your stability ball can help strengthen core muscles and improve balance. Try these exercises during short breaks or when you need a quick energy boost:

Seated Bounces: Gently bounce up and down while maintaining good posture. This can help improve circulation and engage core muscles. Start with 30 seconds and gradually increase the duration as you build stamina.

Pelvic Tilts: Slowly tilt your pelvis forward and backward, focusing on engaging your abdominal and lower back muscles. Perform 10-15 repetitions, holding each tilt for a few seconds.

Seated Marches: Lift your feet alternately off the ground, as if marching in place. This helps improve balance and core strength. Aim for 20-30 marches, alternating legs.

Side-to-Side Rolls: Gently roll the ball from side to side, maintaining balance and engaging your oblique muscles. Perform 10-15 rolls to each side, focusing on controlled movements.

Scientific Findings

A 2009 study in the *Journal of Occupational and Environmental Hygiene* found that stability ball users showed **greater trunk motion and energy use** than chair users, though prolonged sitting caused increased discomfort.[11]

A 2016 *Human Factors* study found **increased activity but no major pain reduction**, reinforcing that variety — not any one tool — is key to spinal health.[12]

***

Chapter Quick Summary – 10 Keys to Safe and Effective Stability Ball Use

Choose the right size for your height.

Begin with 15–30 minute sessions.

Maintain upright posture and relaxed shoulders.

Take standing breaks hourly.

Alternate with a traditional chair.

Perform light bounces and tilts to engage your core.

Use a base for safety during long tasks.

Combine with stretching and movement breaks.

Listen to your body — adjust or rest if sore.

Treat the ball as part of a varied posture plan.

Looking Ahead

You've now explored three innovative seating options — saddle stools, kneeling chairs, and stability balls — each designed to restore movement to the modern workspace. Next, in Chapter 11, we'll shift focus to **ergonomic accessories and small adjustments** that enhance comfort and help fine-tune your daily environment.

Chapter 11

Ergonomic Accessories

Fine-Tuning Your Workspace

Once your chair, desk, and posture are correctly set up, it's time to enhance comfort with accessories that fine-tune your ergonomic environment. Small additions — like a footrest, wrist rest, or document holder — can make a substantial difference to how your body feels at the end of the day.

Ergonomic accessories don't just add comfort; they **help prevent strain** by supporting neutral posture, promoting movement, and reducing pressure on key joints. The right tools transform a standard workspace into one that truly supports your health.

Be aware that the process of optimizing your workspace is ongoing. As your body and work habits change over time, you may need to reassess and readjust your ergonomic setup.

Arms and wrists:

Keyboard tray

Ergonomic keyboard and mouse

Wrist support pads

Neck and Head:

Document holder

Hands-free headset

Noise-cancelling headphones

Feet and Legs:

Footrest

Anti-fatigue mat

Low Back:

Wobble Cushion

Posture Wedge

Lumbar Cushion

Chapter 12

Keyboard Tray

A keyboard tray is an essential component for achieving good ergonomics in your workspace. It allows you to position your keyboard and mouse at the optimal height and angle, reducing strain on your wrists, arms, and shoulders during extended periods of computer use.

Benefits of Using a Keyboard Tray

Proper Wrist Alignment: A keyboard tray helps maintain a neutral wrist position, which is crucial for preventing repetitive strain injuries such as carpal tunnel syndrome. By allowing you to adjust the height and tilt of your keyboard, you can ensure that your wrists remain straight and relaxed while typing, rather than bent at an awkward angle.

Customizable Positioning: Most keyboard trays offer a range of adjustments, including height, tilt, and swivel. This flexibility enables you to find the most comfortable position for your individual body type and working style. You can easily switch between positive, neutral, and negative tilt angles to reduce fatigue and promote better posture throughout the day.

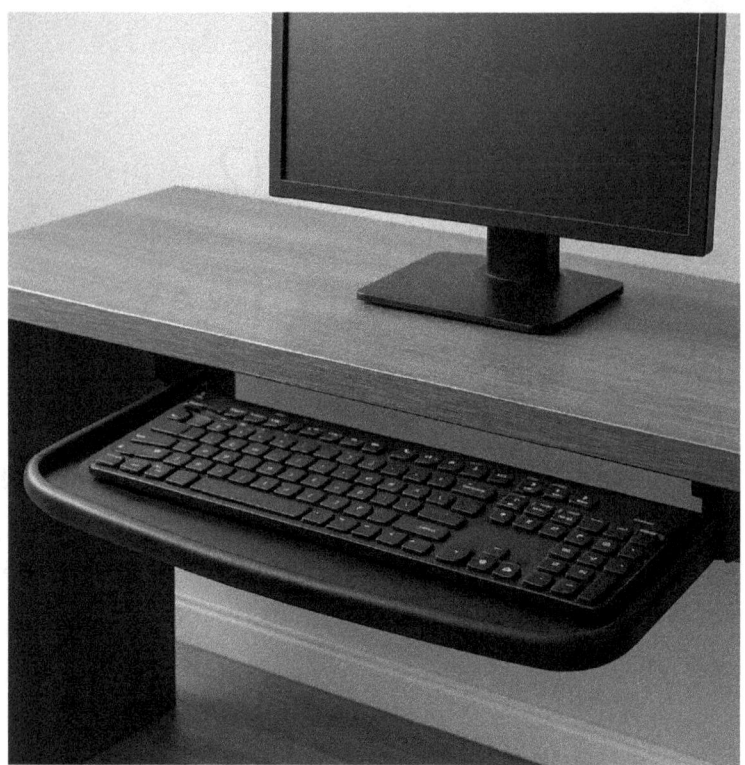

Figure 13 - Keyboard tray below the desktop.

Space-Saving Design: By moving your keyboard and mouse off the desk surface, a keyboard tray frees up valuable workspace. This extra room can be used for other tasks or simply to create a cleaner, more organized environment, which can contribute to improved focus and productivity.

Improved Posture: When your keyboard is positioned correctly, it encourages better overall posture. You're less likely to hunch over your desk or reach awkwardly for your input devices, which can help prevent back, neck, and shoulder pain associated with poor ergonomics.

Increased Comfort for Standing Desks: If you use a standing desk, a keyboard tray becomes even more valuable. It allows you to maintain proper ergonomics whether you're sitting or standing, ensuring that your arms and wrists are always at the right height.

Choosing a keyboard tray

When selecting a keyboard tray, consider factors such as:

Size: Ensure the tray is large enough to accommodate both your keyboard and mouse comfortably.

Adjustment Range: Look for a tray with a wide range of height and tilt adjustments to suit your needs.

Stability: Choose a sturdy tray that will not wobble or sag under use.

Installation: Consider whether you need a clamp-on model or one that needs more permanent installation under your desk.

Chapter 13

Ergonomic Keyboard and Mouse

An ergonomic keyboard and mouse are essential tools for maintaining proper posture and reducing strain during extended computer use. These devices are designed to promote a more natural hand and wrist position, which can help prevent repetitive strain injuries and improve overall comfort.

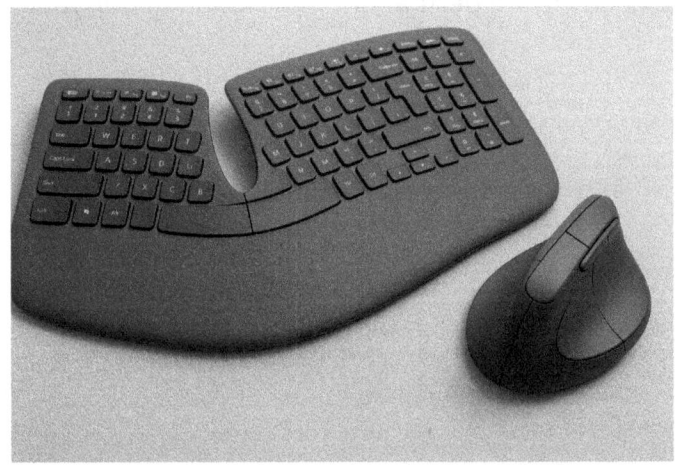

Figure 14 – Using an ergonomic keyboard and vertical mouse helps wrist alignment

Ergonomic Keyboard

Ergonomic keyboards come in various designs, but they all share the goal of reducing wrist strain and promoting a more natural typing position.

Some common features include:

Split design: The keyboard is divided into two sections, allowing for a more natural shoulder-width positioning of the hands.

Curved or contoured surface: This design helps to reduce the need for wrist rotation and extension.

Adjustable tilt: Users can customize the angle of the keyboard to suit their personal needs and preferences.

Wrist rest: Many ergonomic keyboards include a built-in or attachable wrist rest to support the hands and reduce strain.

Using an ergonomic keyboard may require an adjustment period, but many users report reduced pain and discomfort after making the switch.

Ergonomic Mouse

An ergonomic mouse is designed to fit the natural contours of the hand and promote a more relaxed grip. Key features often include:

Vertical or angled design: This encourages a "handshake" position, which reduces forearm twisting and wrist strain.

Thumb support: Many ergonomic mice have a dedicated area for the thumb to rest, promoting a more relaxed grip.

Adjustable sensitivity: Users can fine-tune the mouse's responsiveness to suit their needs and work environment.

Programmable buttons to reduce repetitive movements.

When selecting an ergonomic mouse, it is important to choose one that fits your hand size and preferred grip style for the most comfort and effectiveness.

Chapter 14

Wrist Pads

Ergonomic wrist support pads are essential accessories designed to promote proper wrist positioning and reduce strain during extended periods of computer use. These pads are typically placed in front of the keyboard or mouse, providing a cushioned surface for the wrists to rest on while typing or using a mouse.

Benefits of Ergonomic Wrist Support Pads

Improved Wrist Alignment: By elevating the wrists slightly, these pads help maintain a more natural and neutral position of the wrist joint. This alignment reduces the risk of compression on the median nerve, which runs through the carpal tunnel in the wrist, potentially preventing conditions like carpal tunnel syndrome.

Reduced Muscle Fatigue: The padded surface offers comfort and support, minimizing the effort required to hold the hands and wrists in position. This can significantly decrease muscle fatigue in the forearms and hands during long work sessions.

Enhanced Comfort: The soft, cushioned material of wrist support pads provides a comfortable resting place for the wrists, making extended computer use more pleasant and less physically taxing.

Improved Circulation: By promoting better wrist positioning and reducing pressure points, these pads can help maintain proper blood flow to the hands and fingers, which is crucial for long-term hand health and comfort.

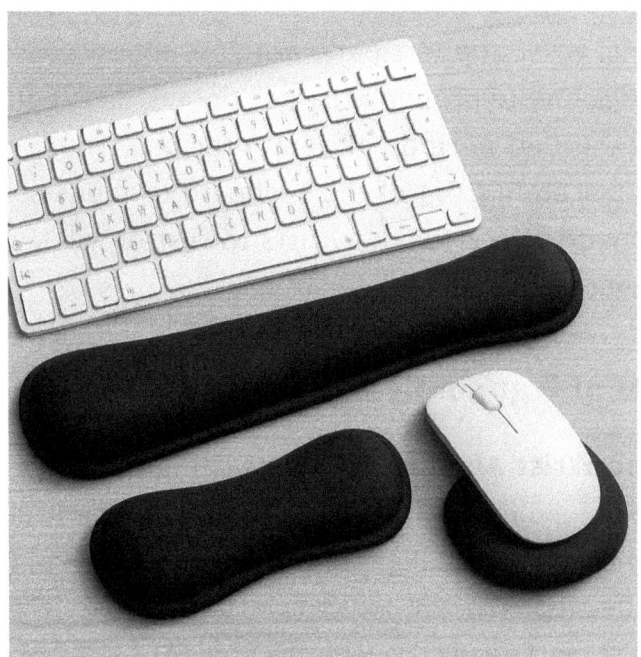

Figure 15 – Wrist support pads help maintain a neutral wrist position

Proper Use of Wrist Support Pads

To maximize the benefits of ergonomic wrist support pads:

Position the pad directly in front of your keyboard or mouse. Rest your wrists lightly on the pad while typing or using the mouse, avoiding excessive pressure.

Maintain good overall posture, with your shoulders relaxed and elbows at approximately a 90-degree angle.

Take regular breaks to stretch and move your wrists and hands.

Choosing the Right Wrist Support Pad

Consider the following features:

Material: Look for pads made from memory foam, gel, or other soft, supportive materials that conform to your wrist shape.

Size: Ensure the pad is wide enough to accommodate your keyboard or mouse and fits comfortably in your workspace.

Non-slip base: A stable, non-slip bottom prevents the pad from sliding during use, maintaining its ergonomic benefits.

Chapter 15

Document Holder

A document holder helps reduce neck strain and eye fatigue by positioning documents at eye level and in line with your computer screen. This alignment minimizes the need for constant head movement between the document and the screen, creating neck and eye strain.

Benefits of Using a Document Holder

Reduces neck strain: By elevating documents to eye level, you minimize the need to look down repeatedly, which can cause tension in the neck muscles.

Improves posture: Proper document placement encourages a more upright sitting position, promoting better overall posture and reducing the risk of back pain.

Enhances productivity: With documents easily visible and accessible, you can work more efficiently, reducing the time spent searching for information or adjusting your position.

Decreases eye strain: Placing documents at a similar distance and angle to your screen helps maintain consistent focus, reducing the strain on your eyes from constant refocusing.

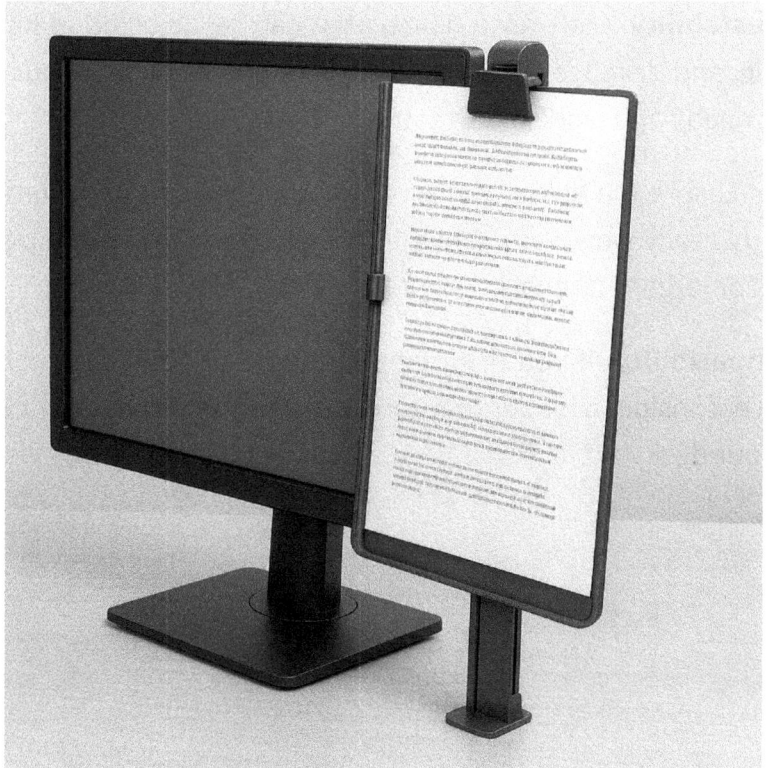

Figure 16 – Correct positioning of document holder

Proper Placement of Your Document Holder

For optimal ergonomics, position your document holder:

At the same height and distance as your screen to minimize head movement and maintain a consistent focal point.

Slightly tilted to match the angle of your screen, typically between 15 to 30 degrees from vertical.

Choosing the Right Document Holder

When selecting a document holder, consider the following factors:

Adjustability: Look for a holder that can be adjusted in height, angle, and distance from your screen to accommodate your specific needs and workstation setup.

Size: Ensure the holder can accommodate the size of documents you typically work with, whether they're standard letter-size papers or larger materials.

Compatibility: If you use many monitors or have limited desk space, consider a holder that can attach to your monitor or clamp to your desk.

Chapter 16

HEADSET

Hands-free headsets are a low-cost, high-benefit addition to the workplace. They play a crucial role in maintaining proper neck and shoulder alignment.

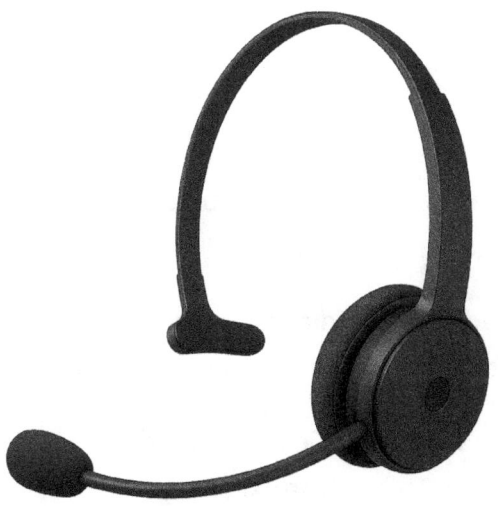

Figure 17 – Hands-free headset reduces neck and shoulder strain. Ideal for frequent callers and virtual meetings

By allowing users to communicate hands-free, headsets eliminate the need to cradle a phone handset between the ear and shoulder. This can lead to chronic neck strain and discomfort from prolonged, repetitive phone use.

Choosing the right headset

When selecting a headset for ergonomic purposes, consider the following factors:

Weight: Opt for lightweight models to minimize strain on your neck and head. Heavier headsets can cause fatigue and discomfort, especially during extended use. Look for headsets made from lightweight materials such as reinforced plastics or lightweight metals.

Fit: Choose a headset that fits comfortably and securely. An ill-fitting headset may cause you to adjust your posture frequently, negating the ergonomic benefits.

Adjustable headbands and ear cushions can help achieve a customized fit for different head sizes and shapes.

Microphone positioning: Select a headset with an adjustable microphone boom. This feature allows you to position the microphone close to your mouth without having to strain your neck or alter your natural speaking posture.

Wireless vs. wired: Wireless headsets offer greater freedom of movement, allowing the user to maintain proper posture while walking or stretching during calls. However, ensure that the battery life is sufficient for a full workday to avoid interruptions.

Sound quality: Audio clarity helps reduce the need to strain or lean forward to hear, which can compromise neck posture. Some headsets have noise-cancelling features to improve audio clarity in noisy office environments.

Compatibility: Ensure the headset is compatible with your existing phone system or computer software.

By implementing ergonomic headsets in the workplace, you can significantly reduce the risk of neck-shoulder strain injuries and improve your overall comfort and productivity.

Chapter 17

Noise-Cancelling Headphones

Noise-cancelling headphones have become an invaluable tool for enhancing workplace concentration. These advanced audio devices use sophisticated technology to detect and counteract ambient sounds, creating a more focused environment for the user.

By employing active noise control, noise-cancelling headphones generate sound waves that are precisely out of phase with the incoming noise, effectively neutralizing it before it reaches the ear.

Benefits of noise-cancelling headphones

Improved focus: By reducing distracting background noise, these headphones allow employees to concentrate more deeply on their tasks. This is particularly useful in open plan offices or shared workspaces where conversations, phone calls, and other ambient soundscan be constant disruptions.

Increased productivity: With fewer auditory distractions, workers can finish tasks more efficiently and with greater accuracy. The ability to maintain uninterrupted focus for longer periods often leads to higher quality work output.

Stress reduction: Constant exposure to noise can be a significant source of stress in the workplace. Noise-cancelling headphones provide a sense of calm and control over your auditory environment, potentially lowering stress levels and improving overall well-being.

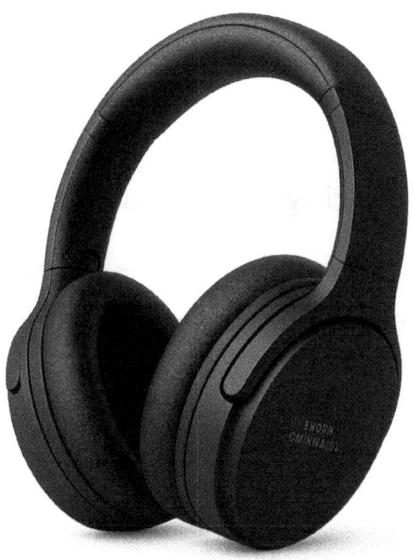

Figure 18 - Noice-cancelling headphones help block background noise

Enhanced privacy: In addition to blocking out external noise, these headphones can also prevent others from overhearing confidential conversations or sensitive information, which is crucial in many professional settings.

Versatility: Many noise-cancelling headphones offer the option to play music or white noise, further customizing the auditory experience to suit individual preferences and work styles.

Choosing headphones

When selecting noise-cancelling headphones for workplace use, consider factors such as comfort for extended wear, battery life for all-day use, and compatibility with various devices used in your work environment.

Some models also feature adjustable noise cancellation levels, allowing users to customize the degree of ambient sound reduction based on their surroundings and personal preferences.

Many modern noise-cancelling headphones include features like transparency mode, which allows users to quickly tune into their surroundings when necessary, without removing the headphones.

Chapter 18

Footrest

A footrest is an essential component of an ergonomic workstation setup, providing many benefits for comfort and health. When properly positioned, a footrest can significantly improve posture, reduce lower back strain, and enhance overall circulation.

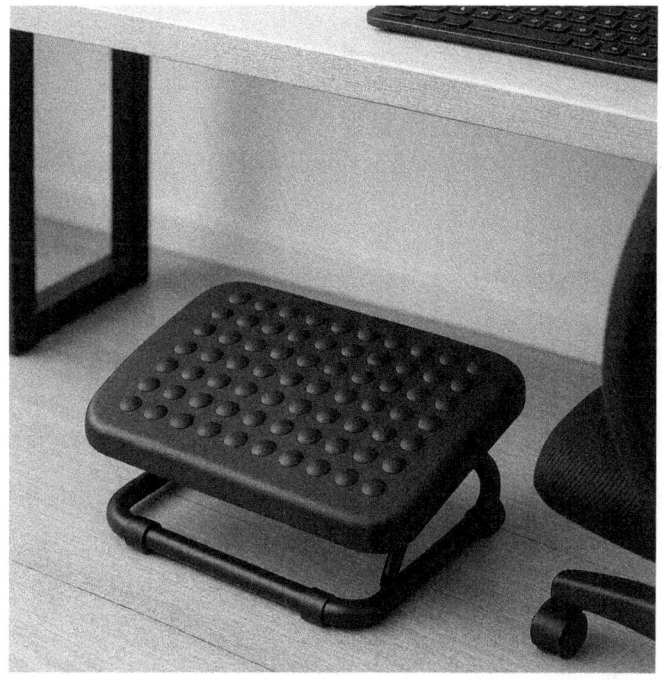

Figure 19 – A footrest supports the feet

Benefits of Footrests

Improved posture: By supporting your feet, a footrest helps maintain proper spinal alignment, reducing the tendency to slouch or lean forward. This improved posture can reduce pressure on your lower back and neck, potentially reducing the risk of developing chronic pain or discomfort associated with prolonged sitting.

Reduced lower back strain: When your feet are properly supported, it helps distribute your body weight more evenly, reducing the load on your lower back. This can be particularly useful for individuals who experience lower back pain or discomfort during extended periods of sitting.

Enhanced circulation: Elevating your feet slightly with a footrest can promote better blood flow in your legs and feet. This improved circulation can help reduce swelling, fatigue, and the risk of developing varicose veins, especially for those who sit for long periods.

Increased comfort: A footrest provides a stable surface for your feet, preventing them from dangling or resting on uncomfortable surfaces. This added comfort can help reduce fidgeting and restlessness, potentially improving focus and productivity.

Customizable support: Many footrests offer adjustable heights and angles, allowing you to customize the support to your specific needs and preferences. This adaptability ensures that you can maintain proper ergonomics regardless of your height or desk configuration.

Proper Positioning of Footrest

Place the footrest under your desk, ensuring it's at a height that allows your feet to rest comfortably while maintaining a 90-degree angle at your knees and hips.

Chapter 19

Anti-Fatigue Mat

An anti-fatigue mat is an essential accessory for standing desk users. These specialized mats are designed to reduce discomfort and fatigue associated with prolonged standing.

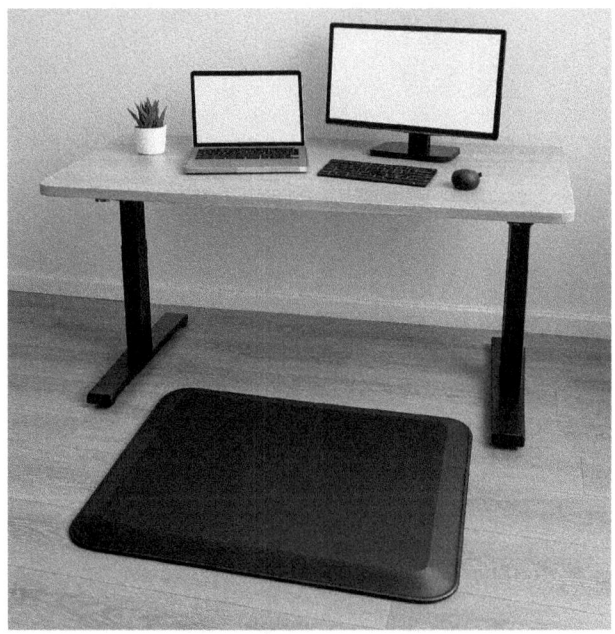

Figure 20 – Anti-fatigue mats reduce standing pressure on joints

Anti-fatigue mats provide a cushioned surface that encourages subtle movements of the feet and legs, promoting circulation and reducing muscle strain.

Benefits of Using an Anti-Fatigue Standing Mat

Reduced Fatigue: The mat's cushioning properties help distribute weight more evenly, lessening the strain on your feet, legs, and lower back. This redistribution of pressure allows you to stand for longer periods without experiencing the same level of fatigue you would on a hard floor.

Improved Posture: The slight instability created by the mat's surface encourages small, unconscious movements in your legs and feet. These micro-movements help maintain better posture and prevent the stiffness that often occurs when standing still for extended periods.

Enhanced Comfort: The cushioned surface provides a more comfortable standing experience compared to hard floors. This added comfort can lead to increased productivity and focus.

Increased Circulation: The subtle movements promoted by the mat help stimulate blood flow in your legs and feet, reducing the risk of circulation- related issues that can arise from prolonged standing.

Choosing the Right Anti-Fatigue Mat

When selecting an anti-fatigue mat for your standing desk, consider the following factors:

Size: Ensure the mat is large enough to accommodate your natural standing position and any movements you make while working.

Thickness: A mat between 3/4 inch to 1 inch thick (1.9 to 2.5 cm) typically provides optimal cushioning and support.

Material: Look for durable materials like high-density foam or rubber that can maintain their supportive properties over time.

Surface Texture: Choose a mat with a textured surface to provide extra grip and prevent slipping.

Chapter 20
Posture Wedge

A posture wedge is a simple yet effective tool designed to improve your sitting posture and reduce discomfort associated with prolonged periods of sitting. This ergonomic device is typically made of high-density foam or similar supportive materials and is shaped like a wedge, with a thicker end that tapers down to a thinner edge.

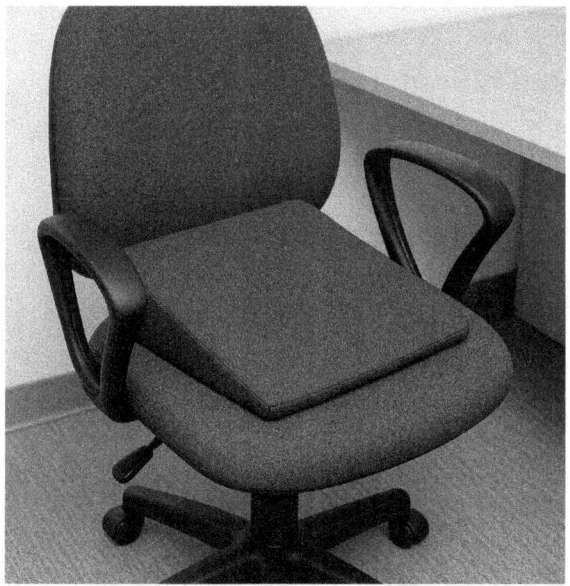

Figure 22 – A posture wedge tilts the pelvis forward, reducing pressure on the low back

How to Use a Posture Wedge

Place the wedge on your chair with the thicker end towards the back.

Sit all the way back on the wedge, allowing your pelvis to tilt forward.

You may need to add a lumbar support, as sitting on the wedge increases the space behind your low back and the chair.

Make sure your chair height is adjusted so your feet are flat on the floor.

How It Works

The posture wedge is placed on your chair or seat with the thicker end towards the back. When you sit on it, the wedge tilts your pelvis forward slightly, which naturally encourages an increased lumbar curve and a more upright spinal alignment.

Benefits of Using a Posture Wedge

Improved Spinal Dynamics: By tilting your pelvis forward, the wedge helps to maintain the natural curvatures of your spine, reducing strain on your back muscles and vertebrae.

Reduced Lower Back Pain: The improved posture can reduce pressure on the lower back, potentially reducing pain and discomfort associated with poor sitting habits.

Enhanced Core Engagement: Sitting on a wedge needs subtle adjustments in your core muscles to maintain balance, which can lead to improved core strength over time.

Increased Comfort During Extended Sitting: The wedge adds extra cushioning to the seat, which helps reduce compression on the low back. Many users report feeling more comfortable during long periods of sitting, such as at work or while driving.

Portable and Versatile: Posture wedges are lightweight and can be easily moved between different chairs or taken with you when traveling.

Chapter 21

Wobble Cushion

Wobble cushions are dynamic seating tools designed to promote active sitting and improve posture. These inflatable discs, typically made of rubber or PVC material, create an unstable surface that engages core muscles and encourages subtle movement while sitting.

How to Use a Wobble Cushion

To use a wobble cushion effectively, place it on your chair seat and sit on it with your feet flat on the floor.

Start with short periods of use, gradually increasing the duration as you become more comfortable with the relative instability.

It's important to maintain good posture while using the cushion, keeping your shoulders relaxed and your spine in a neutral position.

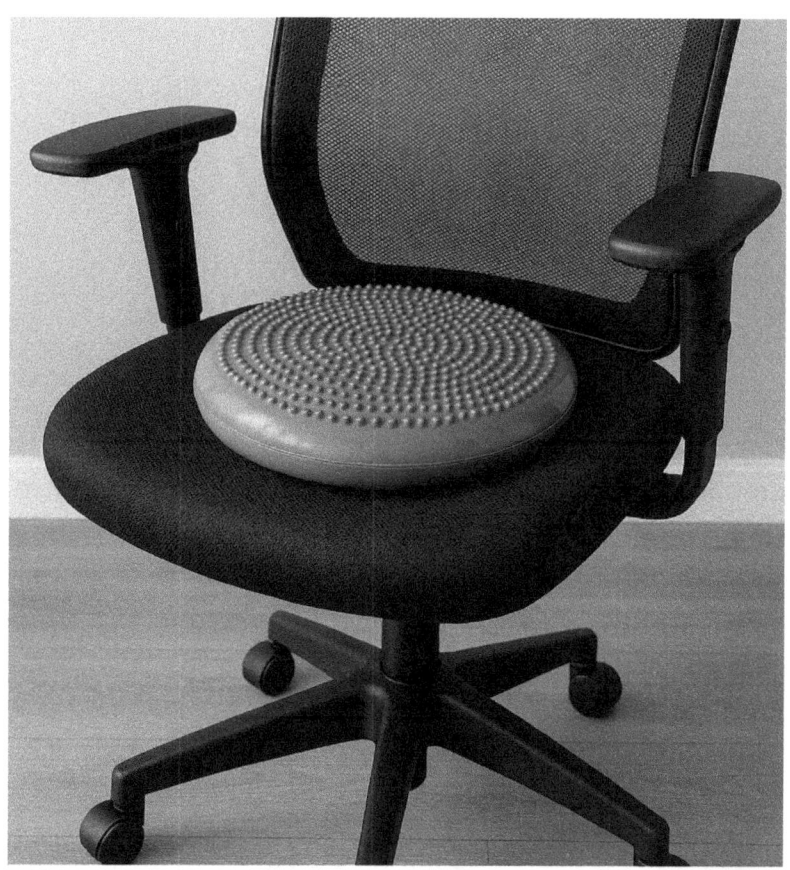

Figure 21 – A wobble cushion reduces static posture fatigue

Chapter 22

Lumbar Cushion

A lumbar support cushion is an essential accessory for maintaining proper posture and alleviating discomfort while sitting for extended periods. This ergonomic device is designed to fit the natural curve of your lower back, providing crucial support to the lumbar region of your spine.

By promoting *proper spinal alignment,* the cushion can significantly reduce the risk of developing or exacerbating lower back pain, a common issue for those who spend long hours seated at desks or in vehicles.

The cushion's design typically features a contoured shape that fits snugly against the lower back, filling the gap between the chair and the inward curve of the lumbar spine. This support encourages users to sit with *improved posture.*

Many lumbar support cushions are made from memory foam or other high-density materials that offer a balance of firmness and comfort. These materials conform to the user's body shape while providing *consistent support,* ensuring that the cushion remains effective throughout extended periods of use.

Portability is another key advantage of lumbar support cushions. Their compact size and lightweight nature make them easy to transport between different seating environments, such as from office chairs to car seats or even airplane seats during travel.

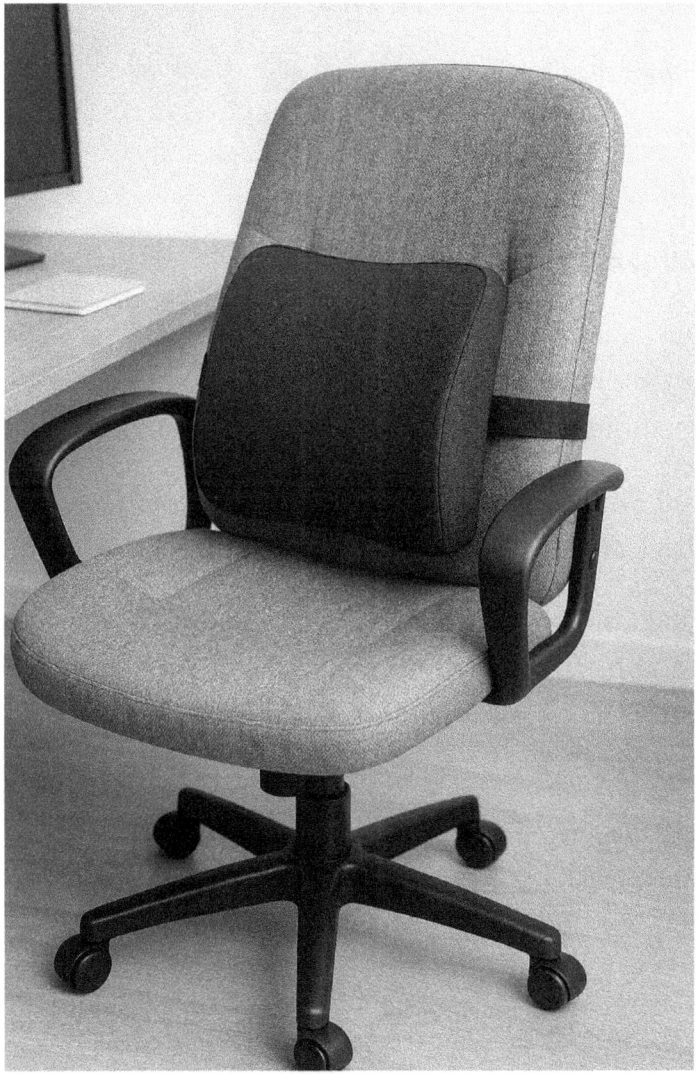

Figure 23 – Lumbar cushions provide targeted lower back support and maintain lumbar curve.

Benefits of Lumbar Cushions

Regular use of a lumbar support cushion can lead to many benefits:

- *Reduced lower back pain* and discomfort.

- *Improved posture* and spinal alignment.

- *Decreased muscle fatigue* in the back and core.

Choosing a Lumbar Cushion

Lumbar cushions come in various shapes and sizes, ranging from compact lumbar rolls to full-length back supports. When selecting the right lumbar support cushion, consider the following factors:

Size and Fit: Ensure the cushion fits comfortably against your lower back and aligns with the natural curve of your spine.

Material: Common materials include memory foam, gel-infused foam, and high-density foam. Memory foam contours to your body for personalized support, while gel-infused options offer cooling properties.

Adjustability: Look for cushions with adjustable features, such as straps or removable inserts, to customize the fit and support level according to your needs.

Attachment mechanisms: Cushions equipped with straps or other attachment methods can be secured to chairs, preventing slippage and maintaining consistent support during use.

Cover and Maintenance: Opt for cushions with removable and washable covers made from breathable fabrics to ensure hygiene and comfort over time.

Portability: If you plan to use the cushion in multiple settings (e.g., office, car, home), consider lightweight and portable designs for ease of transport.

By evaluating these factors, you can select a lumbar cushion that enhances comfort, supports proper posture, and alleviates lower back discomfort during prolonged sitting.

Chapter 23

Conclusion – Living And Working In Alignment

Working from home remotely or in a hybrid arrangement have reshaped how we live, move, and connect. Yet the foundation of every productive workday remains the same — a body that feels supported, balanced, and free from pain.

The principles in this guide are not just about furniture or posture; they're about awareness. When you understand how your workspace influences your body, you can make small, deliberate changes that transform comfort, focus, and long-term health.

Ergonomics is not a one-time setup. It's a daily practice of tuning in — noticing how you sit, how often you move, and how your environment supports you. Over time, those mindful adjustments become habits that strengthen both body and mind.

Your home office can be more than a place to work. It can be a space that restores energy, enhances concentration, and supports wellbeing for years to come.

Work smart. Sit right. Feel great.

Annotated Bibliography

1. Owl Labs. (2022). State of Remote Work. Retrieved from

Annotation: This report provides statistics on remote and hybrid work trends, setting the stage for why ergonomic solutions are increasingly relevant. It emphasizes the scale of the shift in work environments and validates the book's relevance in today's professional landscape.

2. Chen, S. (n.d.). Quote attributed to Dr. Samantha Chen, Ergonomics Specialist.

Annotation: This quote emphasizes the dual nature of remote work—offering flexibility while demanding greater personal responsibility for health. While the original source is unspecified, the quote underscores a key message in the book: that ergonomics must evolve alongside modern work environments.

3. LinkedIn News. (2022, October). Hybrid work wellness: How to support employees wherever they work. Retrieved from

Annotation: This article outlines how Orion Tech, a mid-sized global tech company, addressed wellness challenges during its transition to hybrid work. Facing rising stress and declining engagement, the company implemented a wellness program that included virtual mental health resources, gratitude-based peer engagement, wellness events, and manager-driven support initiatives. After six months, they reported a 35% increase in employee engagement.

4. American Chiropractic Association. (2021). Impact of the COVID-19 Pandemic on Musculoskeletal Health.

Annotation: This study reports a sharp rise in musculoskeletal complaints such as back and neck pain during the shift to remote work, reinforcing the book's argument that home-based work setups have significant consequences for physical health. It validates the need for ergonomic interventions as people adapt to long-term remote work.

5. Levine, J. A. (n.d.). "Sitting is the new smoking" — Public commentary on sedentary behavior. Mayo Clinic–Arizona State University Obesity Solutions Initiative.

Annotation: Dr. Levine's now-famous quote underscores the severity of sedentary lifestyles as a public health concern. The statement encapsulates the urgency of addressing prolonged sitting—a key issue the book aims to resolve through ergonomic strategies.

6. Autodesk Inc. (2012). Workplace Ergonomics Initiative: Company Case Study on Ergonomic Seating and Productivity. San Francisco, CA.

Annotation: This internal case study from Autodesk demonstrates the measurable benefits of investing in ergonomic seating and employee education. The reported improvements in back pain, absenteeism, and productivity support the book's message that ergonomic interventions yield both health and economic returns.

7. University of Leicester. (n.d.). Standing More at Work Could Burn 30,000 Extra Calories a Year.

Annotation: This study quantifies the caloric and metabolic benefits of standing more frequently during the workday. It strengthens the book's case for incorporating sit-stand routines and encourages readers to adopt small changes that produce long-term health gains.

8. Journal of Occupational Health. (2021). Effects of Sit-Stand Work Routines on Lower Back Pain and Productivity Among Office Workers.

Annotation: This study provides empirical evidence for the benefits of alternating between sitting and standing during the workday. It supports the book's recommendations for sit-stand desks and reinforces the broader theme that posture variation can reduce back pain and enhance well-being.

9. Pronk, Nicolaas P., et al. "Reducing Occupational Sitting Time and Improving Worker Health: The Take-a-Stand Project, 2011." *Preventing Chronic Disease*, vol. 9, 2012, E154.

Annotation: This study provides compelling evidence on the health benefits of sit-stand workstations in the workplace. By implementing sit-stand desks, participants not only reduced their upper back and neck pain by 54% but also improved their overall mood and decreased sedentary time. The reversal of these benefits upon removal of the desks underscores the importance of sustained ergonomic interventions. This research is particularly relevant for organizations aiming to enhance employee well-being and reduce musculoskeletal complaints associated with prolonged sitting.

10. Garrett, Gregory, et al. "Call Center Productivity Over 6 Months Following a Standing Desk Intervention." *IIE Transactions on Ergonomics and Human Factors*, vol. 4, no. 2-3, 2016, pp. 188-195.

Annotation: This study provides empirical evidence on the impact of stand-capable workstations on employee productivity in a call center environment. Over a six-month period, employees who used adjustable desks that allowed them to alternate between sitting and standing demonstrated a 45% increase in productivity compared to those with traditional seated desks.

11. Journal of Occupational and Environmental Hygiene. (2009). Comparison of Trunk Motion and Energy Expenditure Between Stability Ball and Office Chair Use.

Annotation: This study found that using a stability ball as a chair increases trunk movement and energy use compared to a traditional reported increased discomfort during prolonged use, suggesting that stability balls may not be suitable for everyone or for all-day use.

12. Human Factors. (2016). The Effects of Alternative Workstation Seating on Lower Back Discomfort and Physical Activity.

Annotation: This study compared traditional chairs, stability balls, and standing desks. While alternative seating increased physical activity, it did not significantly reduce lower back discomfort in the short term. The findings underscore the importance of individual variability and support the book's message about personalized ergonomic solutions.

Author

Dr. Susan Jameson, Chiropractor

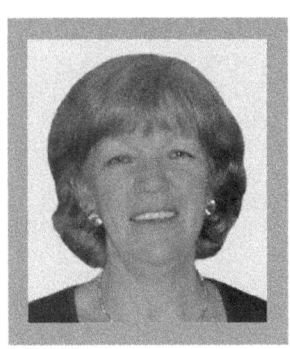 Dr Susan Jameson is a chiropractor, ergonomics educator and workplace wellness advocate dedicated to helping people work, move, and live with less pain. With decades of clinical experience supporting desk-bound office workers, remote professionals and students, she teaches evidence-based strategies that make healthier posture and daily movement achievable for everyone.

Whether you're a professional, student, or freelancer, Dr. Jameson's expert insights aim to help you reduce discomfort, boost energy and feel better every day.

Learn more at: https://betterbacksolutions.com.au

ALSO IN THIS SERIES

Discover other books in the Ergonomic Wellness Series

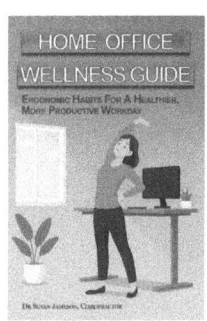

Home Office Wellness Guide: Ergonomic Habits For A Healthier, More Productive Workday

Learn how small, consistent ergonomic and lifestyle habits can restore energy, reduce fatigue, and help you work with greater comfort and clarity.

Scan the QR code to see the book in your preferred bookstore

or visit:

https://books2read.com/u/4ADrWo

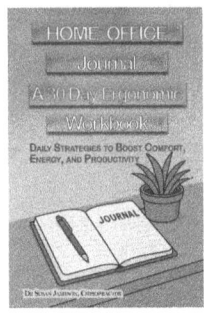 **Home Office Journal – A 30-Day Ergonomic Workbook – Daily Strategies To Boost Comfort, Energy And Productivity**

A 30-day ergonomic reset designed to improve comfort, increase energy, and boost productivity for home office and remote workers.

 Scan the QR code to see the book in your preferred bookstore or visit:

https://mybook.to/HomeOfficeJournal

Leave A Review

Thank you for reading **Home Office Handbook: Ergonomic Solutions for Back Pain (Second Edition)**

If you found this book helpful, please take a moment to leave a review. Your feedback makes a real difference, and helps others discover the book.

Thank you!

Scan QR Code to go to book page.

Scroll down to the review section to leave your review.

Or visit: https://books2read.com/u/mgB2oX

www.ingramcontent.com/pod-product-compliance
Lightning Source LLC
Chambersburg PA
CBHW071719020426
42333CB00017B/2327